WOMEN'S HEALTH AND CORPORATE MARKETING

This compelling collection of essays examines how historically significant marketing schemes have profoundly impacted women's health and healthcare across the world.

Written by scholars and activists from a range of disciplines, including law, sociology, and the health sciences, the book spotlights a range of products that have had a damaging impact on women's health, laying bare the values and assumptions engrained within the marketing campaigns that promoted them. Examples include the advertisement of household and personal care products that expose users to toxic chemicals, empowerment messaging to persuade women to use tobacco products in low- and middle-income countries, and the deceptive marketing of benzodiazepines and opioids that disproportionately impacts women and their families.

A powerful critique of the unethical and paternalistic approach of some corporations, this book will find readers among students taking courses in Public Health, Allied Health, Gender Studies, Sociology, and beyond, as well as interested professionals and lay readers.

Mary Hunter is an Assistant Clinical Professor at the University of California San Francisco School of Nursing. Her current research focuses on the prescription of potentially inappropriate medications associated with cognitive decline in women, including estrogen, benzodiazepines, and opioids. As a nurse practitioner who has dealt with problems related to addiction both in and out of a clinical environment, she is motivated by the fact that drug dependence is everywhere, and finding appropriate treatment for victims is problematic.

WOMEN'S HEALTH AND CORPORATE MARKETING

Our Bodies, Their Business

Edited by Mary Hunter

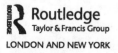

Routledge
Taylor & Francis Group

LONDON AND NEW YORK

Cover credit: © Ryan McVay/Getty Images

First published 2025
by Routledge
4 Park Square, Milton Park, Abingdon, Oxon OX14 4RN

and by Routledge
605 Third Avenue, New York, NY 10158

Routledge is an imprint of the Taylor & Francis Group, an informa business

British Library Cataloguing-in-Publication Data
A catalogue record for this book is available from the British Library

Library of Congress Cataloging-in-Publication Data
Names: Hunter, Mary (Writer on women's health), editor.
Title: Women's health and corporate marketing/edited by Mary Hunter.
Description: London; New York, NY: Routledge, 2025. | Includes
bibliographical references and index.
Identifiers: LCCN 2024011251 (print) | LCCN 2024011252 (ebook) |
ISBN 9781032751603 (hardback) | ISBN 9781032750378 (paperback) |
ISBN 9781003472711 (ebook)
Classification: LCC RA778 .W753 2025 (print) | LCC RA778 (ebook) |
DDC 613/.04244--dc23/eng/20240325
LC record available at https://lccn.loc.gov/2024011251
LC ebook record available at https://lccn.loc.gov/2024011252

ISBN: 978-1-032-75160-3 (hbk)
ISBN: 978-1-032-75037-8 (pbk)
ISBN: 978-1-003-47271-1 (ebk)

DOI: 10.4324/9781003472711

Typeset in Times New Roman
by KnowledgeWorks Global Ltd.

CONTENTS

FOREWORD

Judy Norsigian and Kiki Zeldez, Co-founders of Our Bodies Ourselves

Women's Health and Corporate Marketing: Our Bodies, Their Business is a much-needed, updated review of the many ways that women's health is compromised by corporate interests whose primary objective is maximizing profits. As an organization committed to protesting those instances where the health and well-being of our communities is sacrificed at the altar of the "bottom line," Our Bodies Ourselves welcomes evidence-based critiques of marketing and sales tactics like those in this book.

In an age of escalating commercialism in all sectors of our lives, it is especially apt that we repeatedly underscore the Precautionary Principle of Public Health, which reminds us that the "Absence of Evidence of Harm is not the Same as Proof of Safety." If we don't ask probing questions and don't insist on adequate safety research, we are much more likely to expose ourselves and our communities to avoidable harms. As much of our experience demonstrates, we cannot depend upon corporate interests to take on this critical role. Often, there can be effective collaborations between community groups and government agencies whose mission it is to protect the public's health, and this sometimes entails a "watchdog" function when corporations don't behave responsibly.

A first step in setting out any agenda for evidence-based advocacy is to gather accurate information like the content of this book. Over the years, Our Bodies Ourselves has worked closely with academics and researchers who have helped us identify instances where the profit motive has had a particularly negative impact on women's health. They were often key to developing effective educational campaigns to alert the public, and we see *Women's Health and Corporate Marketing: Our Bodies, Their Business* as a valuable resource in such ongoing efforts of non-profit public interest organizations.

As we reflect back on five decades of educational and advocacy work, the following examples demonstrate well the value of collaborations with academics like those who have authored chapters in this book. We offer these in the spirit of encouraging more such cooperation in the future.

Breast implant safety. The rush to market breast implants—especially silicone-gel implants—well before adequate safety studies were done has resulted in much harm to women. And without the organizing efforts of multiple women's organizations and health groups over many years, it is not clear that any of the more recent actions and warnings of the U.S. Food and Drug Administration (FDA) (for example, the new black-box warning about breast implant-associated anaplastic large cell lymphoma) would have come about. Scientists who worked on exposing these harms were essential to the successful advocacy work of many women's and public health organizations over several decades. (Some of this story is told in the excellent documentary *Absolutely Safe.*)

Pervasive payment incentives in childbearing. Many analyses have pointed to the damage done by the misuse and overuse of routine obstetrical interventions, often encouraged by reimbursement practices in this country. And even after some technologies were determined to be harmful if used routinely—like the internal fetal heart monitor—it took years for mainstream practice to catch up with the evidence. Many factors influence the unacceptably high rate of cesarean section in this country, for example, and the business model governing most systems that offer childbearing services often makes it difficult to align care with best practices. Despite the evidence demonstrating improved birth outcomes with greater access to midwifery care in all settings, it is still difficult to access such care in most communities across the country. And despite clear evidence supporting the benefits of offering VBAC (vaginal birth after cesarean), women seeking an appropriate VBAC often find that this option is totally unavailable in their community.

The multi-billion-dollar fertility industry. Fertility centers and clinics have engaged in potentially harmful practices that go well beyond the appropriate purview of providing good-quality medical care for those people needing services to support family formation. As a result of the insidious role played by the profit motive and dysfunctional reimbursement practices, we now see serious problems with the following: Unethical payment incentives and inadequate informed consent for younger women providing eggs for fertility purposes; far too many implantations of multiple embryos (rather than single-embryo transfers, now pretty much the standard of care in all other industrialized countries); inadequate informed consent, unethical recruitment tactics, and unethical restrictions on gestational mothers ("surrogates") that have led to documentable harms, including deaths; and a public discourse that hides the realities of transnational commercial surrogacy. The work of scholars/colleagues in the assisted reproduction field has been essential to the advocacy work of groups like the Center for Genetics and Society (see www.surrogacy360.org for more history).

Inappropriate drug marketing. Back in the 1970s, groups like the National Women's Health Network and Our Bodies Ourselves protested the unscientific marketing of estrogen products to women of perimenopausal age. Later, the New View Campaign led a major effort to expose the ineffective and potentially harmful drugs promoted for female sexual dysfunction, a term often defined in misleading and inaccurate ways. Despite clever marketing campaigns by the drug industry (e.g., the "Your Voice, Your Wish" website), advocates exposed the distorted "statistics" ("43% of women suffer from some form of sexual dysfunction") and secured warning ads for at least one drug that did finally get FDA approval (flibanserin). This campaign was remarkably successful in raising awareness about flibanserin-related problems and its marginal efficacy.

Since the 1990s, those in the United States have watched direct-to-consumer advertising for prescription drugs proliferate at a rapid pace. In such ads, benefits are often overstated while risks are typically understated. FDA warning letters, if issued, appear *after* the ads run, and corrective ads are rarely required. Withdrawal of an ad is the only penalty for misleading the public this way, so *caveat emptor* now prevails. Chapters in this book continue to alert the public to this persistent challenge. When the public sees ads with famous people claiming that a particular drug helped them, when the scientific evidence doesn't support such claims, information like that found in *Women's Health and Corporate Marketing: Our Bodies, Their Business* will help people achieve a more balanced view.

In her book *The Rise of Viagra: How the Little Blue Pill Changed Sex in America*, sociologist Meika Loe examined the confluence of cultural anxiety, profit motive, and mega-marketing that has made Viagra a bestseller (this and similar drugs are now used by millions of men of varying ages since the drug's introduction in 1998). Books like this helped non-profit organizations such as ours be more effective in our public outreach efforts. Misleading marketing to both consumers as well as medical providers will likely be with us for years to come, so we are grateful to authors like those featured in this book for the resources and insights they offer. We also encourage teachers and advocates who will use *Women's Health and Corporate Marketing: Our Bodies, Their Business* in their course selections to inject some humor whenever they can.

ACKNOWLEDGMENTS

With thorough and persuasive scholarship and leadership, Ruth Malone has inspired students in nursing, sociology, medicine, and pharmacy to question and challenge corporate influence on health and healthcare. When the tobacco epidemic finally ends, Dr. Malone deserves much of the credit. See https://profiles.ucsf.edu/ruth.malone.

We are grateful to everyone who supported our book project. The critiques and suggestions of editors and reviewers have been invaluable. Thank you for *getting it* and for your generosity and time.

INTRODUCTION

Mary Hunter

More than five decades ago, a group of women in Boston, Massachusetts, in the United States (US) decided that a key to improving women's healthcare was listening to each other and sharing what they heard.[1] By publishing the groundbreaking book *Our Bodies, Ourselves*, reliable health information based on a combination of lived experience and vetted science was made widely available. Using the perspectives of a variety of women to inform health education, the practice of medicine, and health policy, the Boston Women's Health Book Collective initiated a historic and enduring women's health movement. By critically examining health practices and policies and their social consequences, this heroic and hard-working group of women expanded the social justice movement.

After undergoing frequent updates and translation into multiple languages, the latest print version of *Our Bodies, Ourselves* was released in 2011.[1] Through its online presence as OurBodiesOurselvesToday.org, the organization continues to educate and advocate for girls, women, and gender-expansive people globally. We are honored that the Board of *Our Bodies Ourselves* has endorsed our project. Our book's subtitle is, of course, a homage.

We are five scholars and activists with backgrounds in journalism, law, sociology, health sciences, patient advocacy, and health policy working to advance social justice for women worldwide. Six topics were chosen for their relevance to the theme of the book, which is *women's health and corporate marketing*. The topics are (1) marketing using racialized and misogynistic messaging and the use of scent to promote household and personal care products that expose users to toxic chemicals; (2) marketing using empowerment messaging to persuade women to use tobacco products, particularly in lower-income and middle-income countries with developing economies; (3) deceptive marketing of

DOI: 10.4324/9781003472711-1

benzodiazepines and opioids that disproportionately impacts women and their families; (4) endometriosis treatment drug marketing that unduly influences treatment guidelines, limits patient options, and adversely impacts fertility outcomes; (5) marketing of disposable menstrual hygiene products using messaging that reinforces the construction of the female body and nature as inferior and discourages the use of reusable products; and (6) agist and deceptive marketing of menopausal hormone therapy to older women, women who bear the greatest burden of disease from long-term use.

Each chapter is an examination of corporate marketing practices that harm women. Some of the world's largest multinational corporations (MCNs) are represented: chemical manufacturers, household and personal care conglomerates, tobacco companies, and pharmaceutical giants. These companies have a legal right to ignore the externalized costs of doing business because the legal structure of every corporation requires only profitability. Corporations have *limited liability* for the harm they cause to individuals and groups, and this constrains legal remedies, such as monetary compensation for damages. Limited liability protection encourages corporations to obfuscate scientific facts, including evidence of harm, and to claim product benefits not supported by science. Corporations are given free license to ignore risks associated with their products and sell sickness to women.

US and Global Corporate Power

Without a corporate legal structure allowing individuals to invest in concert with others and to limit an investor's liability in risky ventures, many ambitious and costly enterprises potentially benefiting society might never be undertaken.[2] Limiting the liability of stockholders to the amount they invested was a key feature of the corporate legal structure from the beginning. Some of the earliest corporations were shipping companies in Britain that brought settlers to America, kept them supplied with food and other necessities, and allowed them to maintain family and business connections.

Before the American Revolution, North America was essentially a group of corporate colonies forced by Britain to supply cheap labor, buy British products, and pay taxes.[2] The legal structure of shared stock companies in the US evolved in response to business developments, political sentiment, and key US Supreme Court justice confirmations. In 1776, in his book *The Wealth of Nations*, Adam Smith critiqued corporations for abusing power, corrupting governments, and oppressing citizens.[3] When the US Constitution was written, the power to grant corporate charters to carry out specific activities during specific periods of time was assigned to the states.[2] Between 1819 and 1886, US Supreme Court rulings eroded limits on corporate power by allowing corporations to own stock in other corporations and claim the legal rights of natural personhood. A US Supreme

Court ruling in 1978 affirmed the right of a corporation to make campaign donations to influence elections.

Because shareholders expect the value of their investments to increase, and liability indemnity is limited to the amount invested by the shareholder, "externalized" costs are shifted to individuals and society.[2] Diagnosis and treatment of emphysema, chronic obstructive pulmonary disease, and various cancers are some of the externalized costs associated with the tobacco, fossil fuel extraction, and automobile industries. Externalized costs associated with the pharmaceutical industry include the potential side effects of drugs, such as lasting physical and mental impairment, life-threatening illness, and death. Cancers caused by exposure to chemicals in personal care products, chemicals used in the maintenance of outdoor environments, and chemicals used in the manufacture and maintenance of indoor finishes and furnishings are other examples of externalized costs. Additional externalized costs are borne by workers producing these products.

Of the 100 largest MNCs in the world (by market capitalization), over half are based in the US.[4] This list includes corporations that manufacture and market the personal care, tobacco, and pharmaceutical products discussed in this book. Other countries with large numbers of MNCs are China, Japan, the United Kingdom, and India. Some economists have argued that corporations collectively hold as much power as nation-states.[5] This may explain why government agencies throughout the world often fail to regulate the production, marketing, and sales of dangerous consumer products or to effectively address associated environmental consequences.

MNCs depend on free trade policies that allow them to shift manufacturing to countries with cheaper labor costs.[2,6,7,8,9,10,11] Much of the job shifting occurs between countries in the Global North, which includes most high-income countries, and countries in the Global South. This offshoring of labor has significant consequences both for workers in high-income countries who lose their jobs and workers in lower-income and middle-income countries who assume the jobs. Studies have shown that many women in the US whose jobs are moved elsewhere are forced to rely on part-time work, lose guaranteed income and benefits, and struggle to maintain a living wage. Women of color are most affected. Women in the Global South who work for MNCs are usually not protected by labor laws common in high-income countries, such as limits on work hours, provisions for safe working conditions, and protections from sexual harassment.

Philosophy, Politics, Policy, and Power

Neoliberalism is an economic philosophy associated with policies of deregulation, globalization, and free trade.[2,6,7] Associated with the work of economists such as Milton Friedman at the University of Chicago and the rise of conservative think tanks funded by corporations, neoliberal theory asserts that business interests should be allowed to flourish without regulation and *The Market* should determine which companies and products become successful.[12] Between the Reagan and Clinton administrations in the US, a neoliberal discourse became hegemonic.[2,6,7] This economic discourse is perceived as undisputed common sense by many voters and elected officials in the US, Europe, and other high-income countries.

A branch of feminist sociology that examines the consequences of shifting manufacturing jobs to the Global South is *transnational feminism*.[9,10,11] To a greater extent than somewhat similar feminist study areas, such as *post-colonial feminism, global feminism,* or *intersectional feminism,* transnational feminism focuses on the political causes of economic and social problems for women. Transnational feminist theory identifies neoliberal political agendas and policies as the root causes of such problems as inadequate working conditions, increased debt burden among workers, and the sexualization of women's work. Transnational feminists advocate for protective conditions for women workers in international trade agreements.

Philosophers and social scientists have written volumes about social processes and their impacts on the health of individuals and groups. Michel Foucault noted that powerful entities create discourses that shape our perceptions and guide our actions.[13] A significant discourse impacting public health is the neoliberalist argument that government regulation of commerce, including regulations to protect the environment and public health, makes the US vulnerable to a socialist takeover.[6,7] A closely related discourse involves the creation of doubt about science.

In their books *Merchants of Doubt* and *The Big Myth*, Naomi Oreskes and Erik M. Conway documented how a fear of government regulation rooted in a fear of socialism and communism motivated prominent scientists to produce scientific papers (underwritten by think tanks supported by politicians promoting neoliberalism) challenging established science.[6,7] Some of the same scientists who produced papers disputing the fact that tobacco causes lung cancer also published papers arguing that fossil fuel production and consumption do not contribute to climate change.

The science establishing causation of lung cancer by tobacco use, as well as causation of climate change by fossil fuel production and consumption, that corporate-funded academics wrote papers to debunk was already settled.[6,7] Peer-reviewed publications had been validated by leading academics and accepted as such by government officials. Claiming "scientific" uncertainty about established medical tobacco science and climate science, these supposedly skeptical academics created doubt in the minds of consumers, politicians, and policymakers. This doubt gave smokers a reason not to quit and drivers an excuse to buy gas-guzzling cars and trucks. These two discourses, namely a neoliberalist resistance to government regulation and a lack of respect for science, are used by corporations to increase their power. Both discourses are evident in marketing schemes discussed in this book.

The Purpose of this Book

The primary purpose of this book is to increase awareness of deceptive corporate marketing by describing several campaigns targeting women. Using a variety of scholarly approaches, the chapters reflect each author's disquiet about a product as well as her professional commitment to address the harms caused by marketing the product. We hope that our diverse examples are useful to readers with their own concerns about corporate influence on health.

A Note on Tone and Style

Because we work and publish in different disciplines, the tone of our writing ranges between personal and informal and neutral and field-specific. Although we each have a personal stake in the research we report, the chapters show variation regarding the incorporation of personal information. We think this tonal variation supports authenticity and accessibility, particularly for readers who share a particular author's experience and background.

Chapter Descriptions with Author Information

Chapter 1 The Stink of Clean

Elizabeth Conway is an environmental health communications expert for Women's Voices for the Earth (WVE), a feminist, women-led, North American environmental organization that specializes in research, education, and advocacy regarding the hazards of toxic chemicals that disproportionately impact women's health. WVE projects have brought attention to the industry's use of scent to target women, potentially putting them at higher risk for adverse outcomes.

Elizabeth holds degrees in history, English, and political science and has her MFA in creative writing from the University of Montana, Missoula. Beth's love of language and the power of message and storytelling characterize her accessible and engaging communication of complex science-laden topics. Her writing for WVE has demonstrated how the use of narratives can strengthen alliances and ignite action in communities of unlikely allies.

Building on previous scholarship exploring misogynistic, classist, and racist biases evident in the history of hygiene in the US, "The Stink of Clean" highlights the critical role fragrance plays in why women purchase cleansing and personal care products. It explores how corporations exploit cultural biases and emotional connections associating fragrance with a false sense of being clean at the expense of health. Capitalizing on women's insecurities about how they smell, the consumer industry has created a demand for products with fragrance, many of which have questionable utility and safety.

This chapter calls attention to a lack of regulation and a dearth of research on the safety of chemicals in intimate care products, including absent US Food and Drug Administration safety oversight of ingredients. Elizabeth cites studies linking the use of intimate care products with increased exposure to toxic chemicals like phthalates and volatile organic chemicals and other studies that suggest direct health impacts, such as an association between douching and pelvic inflammatory disease, and the use of genital powders with ovarian cancer. The chapter emphasizes the disproportionate impact these exposures have on Black and Latina women, who are targeted specifically by marketers. The desire to be "clean," as cultivated by the fragrance industry, clearly causes harm.

Chapter 2 Tobacco Industry Corporate Malfeasance and Women's Rights Violations: Are Human Rights Mechanisms the Antidote?

Kelsey Romeo-Stuppy, Managing Attorney of Action on Smoking and Health (ASH), has worked on global tobacco control since 2013. She leads ASH's program on liability, pursuing criminal and civil cases against the tobacco industry. ASH's human rights program is under her purview; this includes drafting reports and advocating with the United Nations Human Rights Council and other international human rights treaty bodies. ASH has drawn attention to successful marketing campaigns to attract racial minorities and women, campaigns that are increasingly effective worldwide. Kelsey trains advocates to use legal and human rights arguments to further their tobacco control efforts, and she has been a presenter and organizer of public health, tobacco control policy, liability, and human rights events around the world. She also serves on the External Advisory Board for the Center for Tobacco Control Research and Education at the University of California San Francisco. Having published numerous articles in peer-reviewed journals, Kelsey has received praise for her legal writing and advocacy. An article published in the American Bar Association's *International Law News on Tobacco and Human Rights in Latin America* was chosen by another ABA Publication, *GP Solo Magazine*, to be included in a "Best of the ABA" feature issue. Kelsey holds a J.D. from the University of Pittsburgh School of Law, where she also earned a certificate in International and Comparative Law.

The first paragraphs of Kelsey's essay best encapsulate the global tobacco industry's behavior and its conscious decision to exploit women:

For the last century, the tobacco industry has been the epitome of corporate malfeasance. For decades, the tobacco industry withheld important health information, targeted vulnerable groups, and even manipulated the public through bad science. Slowly, the world began to realize the harms of tobacco and the industry's role in furthering the tobacco epidemic. Globally, tobacco control policies have become more widespread and effective, in large part thanks to the "tobacco treaty," the World Health Organization's Framework Convention on Tobacco Control (the WHO FCTC). Tobacco corporations have now been found guilty of racketeering and charged with manslaughter and have been held financially responsible for some of their wrongdoing. It is estimated that nearly 22 million future premature smoking-attributable deaths were averted as a result of strong implementation of demand-reduction measures adopted by countries between 2007 and 2014. And in 2022, for the first time on record, global smoking rates dropped.

Because of these positive steps, many believe that the tobacco epidemic is over. Unfortunately, tobacco corporations are quick to adapt and have changed tactics to target "up and coming markets," chief among them lower- and middle-income countries (LMICs) and women. As George Washington Hill, president of the American Tobacco Company (ATC) from 1925 to 1946, allegedly stated, targeting women "will be like opening a new gold mine right in our front yard."

This chapter examines tobacco marketing targeting women, particularly those in low- and middle-income countries, tracks evolving tobacco use, and outlines innovative strategies to address Big Tobacco's persistent criminal activities, specifically strategies employing human rights mechanisms. Also addressed are related issues that directly impact women and women's rights, including tobacco production, exposure to second-hand smoke, economic development, and environmental impacts.

Chapter 3 Mother's Little Helpers and Opioids: Women, Addiction, and the Legacy of Arthur Sackler

Mary Hunter is an Assistant Clinical Professor at the University of California San Francisco School of Nursing. Her current research focuses on the prescription of potentially inappropriate medications associated with cognitive decline in women, including estrogen, benzodiazepines, and opioids. As a nurse practitioner who has dealt with problems related to addiction both in and out of a clinical environment, she is motivated by the fact that drug dependence is everywhere, and finding appropriate treatment for victims is problematic.

Before earning nursing degrees from UCSF and the University of Washington, Mary obtained a Bachelor's degree in history from Mills College in Oakland, California. As a women's health and adult nurse practitioner, she worked in a variety of settings on the US mainland and Hawaii Island. Her most recent clinical position was in the San Francisco Tenderloin District where she was privileged to provide gender-affirming hormone therapy and primary care to an underserved population that included people struggling with addiction.

This chapter outlines a brief history of drugs used for pain and anxiety, starting with the normalization of laudanum in colonial America, continuing through drug regulatory efforts in the early 1900s and the spectacular rise of the pharmaceutical industry in the mid-1900s. Using the example of Arthur Sackler's innovative advertising career (the success of which effectively set up his brothers to acquire and control Purdue Pharma, the maker of OxyContin), common dishonest pharmaceutical marketing tactics are examined. The chapter subsequently discusses the broad social and health consequences of over-prescription of both benzodiazepines and opioids. Various reasons why women bear the heaviest burden of drug dependence are outlined, as are strategies for treatment.

Chapter 4 Under the Influence: Pharmaceutical Relationships and Their Impact on Endometriosis Care

Heather Guidone is the Surgical Program Director of the Center for Endometriosis Care in Atlanta, Georgia. She is responsible for the management of the Center's multidisciplinary care program and for clinical research and education. Heather's primary focus is on improving outcomes by reducing the time to diagnosis and fighting for equitable access to effective treatments. Heather has long been a champion for endometriosis policy reform, patient-centered care, and education. As an advocate for policy improvement and insurance reform, Heather has testified before state and federal legislatures and co-authored legislation passed by local and national lawmakers. These efforts have included a focus on the effects of systemic racism and the experiences of gender-diverse persons related to delayed diagnosis, lack of patient-centered care, and inappropriate treatment. Through network-building among providers, patient advocates, legislators, and governmental and professional working groups, Heather has strived to ensure stakeholder representation in arenas that encompass the treatment of endometriosis and reproductive health. Her efforts have not only improved outcomes for individual women; she has also significantly increased the awareness of endometriosis as a treatable disease.

Heather's chapter is a critique of the endometriosis disease community as it relates to the industry's hold on many who diagnose, treat, and study the disease.

Although modern medical knowledge, clinical experience, and therapies are ever-evolving, endometriosis remains fundamentally mired in outdated and false assumptions. Treatment "standards" based on misinformation leave those struggling with the disease under-resourced and vulnerable to conflicting information about best practices. Moreover, the field of endometriosis care remains exposed and vulnerable to the potential pitfalls of industry influence.

Heather's chapter meticulously details pharmaceutical industry influence on factors that impact treatment, especially the influence on guidelines and treatment protocols that result in the overuse of drugs and the underutilization of timely surgical intervention. She demonstrates how the industry promotes proprietary drugs through entities that receive corporate funding, including patient support communities and politicians. These promotional efforts are multi-layered, extensive, and non-transparent, and they result in unnecessary pain and hardship for patients, including loss of fertility resulting from the delay of diagnosis and treatment.

From the non-profit setting to research to physicians to policy work to editorial boards to political campaigns, pharma partners' influence across the endometriosis landscape is pervasive. When those who are receiving fiscal compensation from pharma and/or have lent perceived support to a particular product or device in turn create guidelines and policies influencing the already failing standards of care—guidelines that bear an ever-increasing "less laparoscopy, more hormone therapy" sentiment—patients can lose access to appropriate treatment.

Chapter 5 Menstruation Repression Discourse in Advertisements: An Ecofeminist Investigation

Anna Kubovski completed her PhD in the Department of Women's and Gender Studies at the University of Haifa, Israel. Her dissertation examined lived and embodied experiences of menstruators in Israel from an ecofeminist perspective. She studies the intersections between menstruation and environmental quality, ecofeminist theory, women's reproductive health, sexuality, body, media, and consumer culture. Anna is also a workshop facilitator and lecturer in the education department of the Haifa Rape Crisis Center (HRCC).

Anna's chapter describes her extensive analysis of advertisements for menstrual pads and tampons and the impact of these ads on women's perceptions of self and behavior as consumers. Themes developed in the analysis are presented to support her thesis that when a woman is persuaded to use the disposable pads and tampons advertised, she risks distancing herself from her body, experiencing shame, and ignoring physiologic symptoms and signs that could suggest illness.

Analyzing the hidden messages in advertisements reveals that the female body is presented negatively—as inferior, dirty, and smelly. It must be constantly regulated to conform to beauty ideals—clean, dry, fragrant, and fresh. Women internalize these messages and employ them on their bodies; they embody the notion that their bodies are less valuable when menstruating and a source of embarrassment and shame.

In addition, Anna writes about how the use of disposable products harms the environment, and she explains that menstrual hygiene management alternatives, such as menstrual cups and washable pads and underwear, are underutilized as a result of typical advertising of disposable products.

Chapter 6 Hot and Bothered by the Menopause Industry

Mary Hunter, an Assistant Clinical Professor at the University of California San Francisco School of Nursing, decided to pursue a career as a nurse practitioner after savoring the first edition of *Our Bodies, Ourselves* and volunteering for ten years in Planned Parenthood clinics. While working in clinical settings that provided care to women, she became increasingly alarmed and fascinated by the extensive, ubiquitous, and deceptive promotion of hormones. She has centered her research career on the risks of long-term hormone therapy, the meaning of "hormone replacement therapy (HRT)" to users, and its promotion by the menopause industry. The topic of menopausal hormone therapy marketing is introduced with a discussion of the social phenomenon and marketing practice known as *medicalization*. Following this discussion is a short history of the hormone industry, which began when observers noticed an apparent connection between the condition of having testes and aggressive behavior (in roosters). Doctors, all of them male, subsequently engaged in surgical experimentation involving implanting the organs of various mammals in humans, eventually concluding that synthetic hormones should be developed. The chemical synthesis of pharmaceutical hormone preparations was influenced by events related to WWII—who knew? Following the summary of historical events is a description of how the pharmaceutical industry, represented by the North American Menopause Society (whose name was changed in 2023 to The Menopause Society), has persisted for over 20 years to argue that the Women's Health Initiative (WHI), a National Institutes of Health clinical trial, as well as the Million Women Study in the United Kingdom that confirmed WHI's results, produced findings that are "faulty." These two landmark studies, demonstrating that long-term menopausal hormone therapy causes excess disease, seriously threatened the bottom line of the menopause industry, and hormone manufacturers didn't take it lying down. Marketing strategies to sustain a demand for "HRT," by framing it as a disease-prevention and anti-aging drug and by creating doubt about risks in the minds of consumers and healthcare providers, are presented in detail.

Notes

1 Davis K. *The making of our bodies, ourselves: How feminism travels across borders.* Next wave. Duke University Press; 2007: xii.
2 Wiist W. The corporation: An overview of what it is, its tactics, and what public health can do. In: Wiist W, Ed. *Bottom line or public health.* Oxford University Press; 2010:14, 15: chapter I.
3 Smith A. *The wealth of nations.* Fall River Press; 2015
4 Statista. The 100 largest companies in the world by market capitalization in 2023 (in billion U.S. dollars). Statista. 2023. www.statista.com/statistics/263264/top-companies-in-the-world-by-market-capitalization.
5 Babic MH, E, Fitchner, J. Who is more powerful—states or corporations?. https://theconversation.com/who-is-more-powerful-states-or-corporations-99616.
6 Oreskes N, Conway EM. *Merchants of doubt: How a handful of scientists obscured the truth on issues from tobacco smoke to global warming.* First US edition. Bloomsbury Press: 2010.
7 Oreskes N, Conway EM. *The big myth: How American business taught us to loathe government and love the free market.* Bloomsbury Publishing; 2023: ix.
8 Sicchia SR, Maclean H. Globalization, poverty and women's health: Mapping the connections. *Canadian Journal of Public Health—Revue canadienne de sante publique.* January/February 2006; 97(1): 69–71. doi:10.1007/bf03405219.
9 Tambe A, Thayer M. *Transnational feminist itineraries: Situating theory and activist practice.* Duke University Press; 2021: 1. Online resource.
10 Jaggar AM. *Gender and global justice.* Polity; 2014: x.
11 Jaggar AM. Vulnerable women and neo-liberal globalization: Debt burdens undermine women's health in the global South. *Theories of Medical Bioethics.* 2002; 23(6): 425–440. doi:10.1023/a:1021333700894.
12 Friedman M. *Capitalism and freedom.* University of Chicago Press; 1962.
13 Foucault M, Foucault M. *The archaeology of knowledge.* First American edition. World of man. Pantheon Books; 1972.

1

THE STINK OF CLEAN

Elizabeth Conway

It's funny how our senses can determine what we remember. I have three children, ages 13 to 24, and while I can give you a general idea of how each of their births went, those memories are blurred together by C-sections, beautiful newborns, painful weeks of healing, and blissful moments of rest. But then I have a crystal-clear memory of standing behind a classmate in our sixth-grade industrial education class and leaning in closer to his gray sweatshirt—almost until my nose touched his shoulder—because he smelled like the laundry detergent my mom used at home. I couldn't get close enough to that smell. I literally wanted to bury my face in the back of his sweatshirt and take in a deep, calming breath. *Awww, that smells so clean!* Sorry kids, but my memory has shaved away your birth stories to make room for the smell of 12-year-old Luke Ferkinhoff's Tide®-scented gray hoodie.

And then there's Irish Spring® Soap. The minute I smell that green bar forged in what I can only imagine to be lush vegetation from the Cliffs of Moher, I'm back to the gold-and-yellow bathroom in the basement of my grandparents' house in Waseca, Minnesota—my toes wrapped in a shag yellow bathmat. *It smells like a fresh, clean shower!* While I'm sure it wasn't the same bar of soap that was there my entire childhood, I could rely on its presence at every visit as much as I could rely on Grandma Fran serving me mint tea after dinner with however much sugar I wanted.

The fact that the smell of a certain soap or an aroma of detergent brings me such vivid memories is a testament to the power of scent. Few triggers can compete with smell. Smell is the strongest of our memory senses. This has to do with the fascinating fact that our body's smell center is directly connected to the brain—the amygdala and the hippocampus, the regions related to emotion

DOI: 10.4324/9781003472711-2

and memory[1]—essentially the brain's memory center. Which means different scents can impact our emotions and spark memories of old emotions.[2] For me, that seemingly simple smell of a freshly washed gray sweatshirt had nothing to do with that gray sweatshirt. It smelled like comfort and protection and rest and well-being, emotions that encompassed the way my parents made me feel growing up. In short, love. That's powerful.

Companies caught a whiff of this power decades ago. There are entire corporate departments and marketing teams designed specifically to capture and capitalize on our emotional connection to scents. The fragrance industry is one of the largest in the world. In 2021, the global market was valued at $30.6 billion, and growth is expected to be $43.2 billion by 2028.[3] In addition to simple standalone perfumes and colognes, scents are added to diapers and pacifiers, trash bags, children's toys, holiday decorations, and they are put in markers, candles, clothing. They are pumped into hotel rooms and doctors' offices and are found dangling from the rearview car mirror. Scents are added to products to cover up odors, to even create "unscented" products and mask "unwanted" smells. This market saturation suggests that consumers are obsessed with how things smell.

And there are few places where fragrances are more prevalent than in the products we use to *clean* our homes and our bodies—products marketed to keep our homes and bodies healthy. But do they? Keep us healthy, that is?

A simple walk through any local grocery store reveals aisle upon aisle of scented cleaning and hygiene products. Fragrances are often the determining factor in whether or not we decide to purchase a product.[4] While formulas for dish soap, for example, may vary slightly based on brand and function, ultimately the make-up of active ingredients is relatively redundant ... except for the product's signature scent. Toss in a little sensory memory (s*niff-sniff Tide®, home, mom*), and ... *Sold*. In a 2016 international survey conducted by the International Fragrance Association (IFRA) and the European Cleaning Journal (ECJ), fragrance is considered to be one of the most important factors for people when deciding which cleaning products to purchase.[5] Scented products represent 89% of laundry, 79% of surface cleaning, and 99% of dishwashing products.[6] Regarding personal care products, 96% of shampoos, 98% of conditioners, and 97% of hairstyling products contain fragrance.[7] Ninety-one percent of antiperspirants, 95% of shaving products, 83% of moisturizers, and 63% of sunscreens contain fragrance.[8,9]

But the problem is, when we so intimately associate clean with a smell, it's not just about smelling good but rather smelling clean. **And in the United States (US), our relationship with clean is tumultuous at best.**

Targeted marketing is employed to make people want to use certain products, especially in the cleansing products marketed to women. Believing that hygiene is intimately connected with US Americans' deeply rooted historical ideas of racial and sexual purity, author Dana Berthold has argued that racist and misogynistic biases and fears impact daily hygiene routines and purchasing practices.[10] In "Tidy Whiteness: A Genealogy of Race, Purity, and Hygiene," she outlined a definition of cleanliness signified by an ideal of "whiteness" associated with race, wealth, social class, and purity. Corporations apply pressure, particularly on women of color, to meet racist and sexist cultural standards for what it means to be clean.

Berthold is not alone in her argument. Conversations led by many scholars address how this *clean* take on morality has a rocky and damaging relationship with patriarchal values and white supremacy culture.[11,12,13,14] Who can forget that *cleanliness is close to godliness*? This reminder is hand-stitched on a throw pillow in at least one of my great aunts' homes.

And of course, it cannot be ignored that baths and baptisms in multiple religions are literally about "cleansing" the body and soul of sin and restoring purity. In these conversations about what *clean* means, we cannot continue without talking about scents, fragrances, smells. It is undeniable that in our marketplaces *clean* and *scent* go hand in hand. The branding, messaging, and prolific use of distinctive scents to sell cleaning and cleansing products confirm that fragrances play a powerful role and enable a relentless pursuit of cleanliness and purity.

In fact, many of the products we purchase to wash our bodies and clean our homes contain toxic (and unnecessary to product efficiency) chemicals linked to adverse health impacts, including asthma and allergies, cancer, and reproductive harm. Are we worried about protecting our health, or are we worried about being perceived as dirty, unworthy, poor, or impure? After all, fragrance chemicals are often some of the most problematic ingredients used in cleaning[15,16] and personal care products.[17] Across the consumer market, research has shown that over one-third of all chemicals used to make fragrances have been classified as toxic or potentially toxic by scientists throughout the world.[18]

Alexandra Scranton, director of science and research at Women's Voices for the Earth and my colleague, has been studying and watch-dogging the fragrance industry and fragrance safety for nearly two decades. In 2017, she wrote a detailed report, *Unpacking the Fragrance Industry: Policy Failures, the Trade Secret Myth and Public Health*,[19] spotlighting numerous concerning issues about the chemicals the industry has sanctioned for use in fragrances, including the following:

- 190 fragrance chemicals have been assigned the signal word "danger" for their Safety Data Sheet;
- 1,175 fragrance chemicals have been assigned the signal word "warning";
- 44 fragrance chemicals require pictogram GHS06 of skull and crossbones to indicate acute toxicity;
- 97 fragrance chemicals require pictogram GHS08 indicating the chemical is a hazard to human health.[20]

A few specific chemicals used to make fragrances include the following:

- Carcinogens such as styrene, methyl eugenol, pyridine, and BHA;
- Reproductive toxins such as phthalates, lilial, and nonylphenol;
- Neurotoxicants such as xylenes and phenol;
- Skin allergens such as linalool, hexyl cinnamal, geraniol, and HICC.

When all is said and done, at least 1,242 fragrance ingredients (*roughly one-third of all fragrance chemicals currently in use*) are included on one or more authoritative lists of chemicals of concern.[21]

Yet, again and again, these often-toxic scents are employed to sell us health, hygiene, and a sense of being clean. Beyond the cultural and social implications of an attempt to clean ourselves into a particular class, or into a mythical sexual and racial purity, the fact remains, aside from a handful of unicorns, that most fragrance chemicals do not clean and do not improve our health. Instead, they release pollutants into our environment and toxins into our bodies.

Who cares if you're healthy. *Sniff sniff.* I want to know if you're clean. And by the millions, women, particularly women of color, are burdened with the consequences. Consider these few stats about the products we use to clean our homes and bodies:

- In most US households, women drive 70 to 80% of the purchasing decisions.[22] On average, the target audience of brands selling baby products, laundry products, and cleaners is 98% women.[23]
- While gender roles and societal expectations have changed over time, a national study showed that women still complete over 55 to 70% of the housework in the average home[24] and the Economic Policy Institute reported that over 95% of house cleaners are female.[25]
- Latina women make up 46% of the housekeeping and domestic cleaning workers.[26]
- Several widely used chemicals in cleaning products are known toxins linked to reproductive harm, including lower fertility rates and excess rates of birth defects and premature births.[27]
- The salon industry is dominated by women workers. Over 90% of professional hairdressers are women,[28] and according to a study by the UCLA Labor Center and the California Healthy Nail Salon Collaborative, the US nail salon workforce is 81% women (79% are foreign-born, about three-quarters from Vietnam).[29]
- Studies show that professional salon workers have a disproportionate incidence of cancers, neurological diseases, immune diseases, birth defects, reproductive disorders, skin diseases, asthma, and breathing problems linked to chemical exposure at work.[30]

- In the US, the personal care market is valued at over 84 billion.[31] Women on average spend 22% more on personal care products than do men.[32] Women use an average of 12 personal care products daily; men use 6.[33]
- According to Nielsen data, African-Americans spend nearly nine times more than their Caucasian counterparts on hair and beauty.[34] Asian-Americans spend 70% more than the average share of the US population on skincare products.[35]
- A report published by the Silent Spring Institute found that hair products specifically marketed to Black women contained several hazardous ingredients.[36]
- The 2021 *Take Stock* survey of California women found that Black and Hispanic/Latinx women use intimate care products at greater rates than do white women; douche use was particularly higher in Black women than in either white or Latinx/Hispanic women.[37]
- A 2019 study found that women who douched two or more times a month or used "feminine" powder once a month had higher levels of volatile organic compounds (VOCs) in their bodies; VOCs have been associated with respiratory symptoms, cancers, and neurological disorders, as well as adverse reproductive system effects.[38] Another study found that douching was associated with higher levels of the toxic chemical phthalates, which are linked to hormone disruption.[39]

When considering our historic and prevailing sexist and racist obsession with hygiene and purity, these stats should surprise no one (and anger everyone). *And again, driving the purchasing decisions of consumers of these products? Drum roll … fragrance.*

Enjoying a pleasant smell and caring about cleanliness are not wrong-headed aspirations. And a great smell can and should bring us joy. Heck, I buy my body soap because I love its peppermint fragrance. But I would be unwise to let social cues and sensory preferences adversely affect my health and that of my family. Perceptions of cleanliness and health are distorted by compelling fragrances that reinforce marketing messages and convince the public to use certain products to avoid social failure despite health risks.[40]

Wafts of fragrance in personal care products tell us that if we don't smell clean we aren't. That's trouble, and it invites trauma, both to our physical and mental well-being. This connection between fragrance and a sense of being clean can specifically influence "how" and "why" we choose the products we use, overruling even our desires to be healthy.

The Case of a Clean Body

What happens when we confuse smells with clean? Well, scented tampons happen. And vulva and vaginal body washes happen. And so do douches, sprays, wipes, powders, dry shampoos, gels, lubricants, moisturizers, exfoliators, creams, steams with patented "odor eliminating formulas." And "new fresh scents." And "natural scents" designed to "address that not-so-fresh feeling"— at the same time perpetuating the myth that (1) vulvas smell; (2) vulvas are dirty; (3) you are dirty, and ultimately, women are simply dirty. Why? It probably has something to do with menstruation (see scented tampons). And it probably has something to do with purity. Not convinced? Stay with me.

While there are innumerable cleaning products on the market, there are few that can be more directly linked to an obsession with purity, cleanliness, and smell than intimate care products. Also referred to as "feminine hygiene products" and "feminine care products," some items are specifically designed for period and menstrual management. Apparently, some people think we need to use a lot of different products to make our vaginas suitably hygienic, during menstruation or all the time.

Here is a quick summary of the types of products currently on the market that have nothing to do with menstrual management (such as a tampon, menstrual pads, period underwear, or menstrual cup), but rather are designed specifically to use to "care" for the vagina and vulva:

- Douches
- Washes
- Wipes
- Sprays and mists
- Vaginal tightening cream
- Bleaches/lighteners
- Creams
- Deodorant suppositories
- Powders
- Moisturizers
- Hydrating serums
- Lotions
- Steamers
- Exfoliators and scrubs
- Dry shampoos
- Other deodorants (bars, sprays, creams)
- Gels
- Salves
- Lubricants
- And (something new to me) after-sex clean-up sponges.

I'm sure I've missed something. And I'm sure there will be something new and necessary for me to use tomorrow. After all, I have a vagina.

Ignoring the fact that not all people who menstruate or who have a vagina identify as women, the industry overwhelmingly markets these products as "feminine," and almost exclusively targets cisgender women and girls. The industry category for these products—"feminine"—infers that using these products makes each of us more of a "lady." An overwhelming number of these products are specifically marketed as "cleansing" items. In 2021 the global "women intimate care" market was valued at over $28 billion and is estimated to reach close to $46 billion by 2031.[41] Meanwhile, projections for the growth of intimate washes expect a 6.44% increase in shares within the next four years.[42] Projections for 2027 expect global sales of vaginal wipes alone to reach $2.07 billion, up from $154.5 million just a decade earlier.[43]

There are products specifically designed for teens, for tweens, for moms, for menstruators, for pre-sex, post-sex, post-workout, for wellness, and simply for "on-the-go." And new products and product lines continue to saturate the market. For example, in 2021, Vagisil launched a line called "OMV!" that is "designed by teens for teens" and comes in "new Berry Bliss" scent.[44] In the meantime, Summer's Eve now brings us their new "Spa" collection for "Daily Intimate Beauty"[45] and an "Active" line with an "Energizing Acti-Cool Blend" that "cools with a boost of freshness."[46]

Marketing tells us that these products are designed to "clean" and "enhance" vaginas and vulvas. Very few products in this industry category do not use the words "fresh," "refresh," "cleanse," "clean," or "hygiene" to market their product. Some of them claim they will leave us "seductively scented."[47] Some are intended for "Date Night."[48] And almost all of them talk about "odor." Odor odor odor. In fact, many of these products are exclusively about addressing odor. Sprays, deodorants, mists, and (and some powders) do virtually nothing but provide a smell.

Even products specifically made to be "fragrance-free" are clearly marketed as providing "odor protection" or are "odor eliminating." Summer's Eve is the largest manufacturer of vaginal and vulvar-use products (and a company that boasts they "created the feminine care category by putting women first" over 50 years ago[49]). In addition to its scented products, Summer's Eve now also sells "fragrance-free" washes and wipes. These products, guaranteed to protect you from your odors, contain unexplained "Odor-reducing ingredients." Even when it's not about fragrance, it's still about the way you smell. Specifically, about how your genitals smell.

You can claim your womanhood by cleansing yourself, by removing said odor. In the not-too-distant past, Vagisil advertisements gave us permission to be "100% Woman 100% of the Time," but—hold the phone—that's only if you use their Anti-Itch Medicated Wipes.[50] Summer's Eve tells us: "Men have fought for it, battled for it, died for it," so we should show our "V" some love by using their "cleansing wipes and wash."[51] Ultimately, it's all about how sexy you are to men. Lemisol Teen has a "refreshing formula" that is specific for a "Teen Girl's Intimate Hygiene."[52] And VeeFresh—VeeGentle encourages you to "wash away odor and impurities from your most sensitive area."[53]

If you're in need of a dusting of extra purity, you can also use products with the word "baby" in the title: Johnson & Johnson's *Baby* Powder tells us that it will make not only our babies but ourselves "baby-soft"; so go on and "baby yourself"[54] and give your body a feeling it will "never out-grow."[55] (Oh, and while not an intimate care product, let's not forget there's a perfume marketed to women and girls called "Love's Baby Soft" that's been selling this same idea for the past 50 years.)

Why wouldn't we want to care for our bodies? Keep them clean. Keep them fresh, refreshed, re-refreshed, re-re-refreshed and sexy. (But not too sexy, just the right amount of sexy. Just that "feminine" kind of sexy.) The underlying message is that we cannot be any of these things without removing our odor. And, based on the sheer variety of products, vaginas don't just smell, they must really, really, really stink.

Where's the Health?

Where indeed. With all the dizzying and dazzling words and an avalanche of intimate care products, it's easy to miss the fact that the word "health" has a very hard time making it into the conversation. Instead, we get language like "Gynecologist Recommended," "Tested," or "Approved." Approved for what? For your vagina's health? To not give me a rash? To not give me an infection? To cure me of my odor? To clean my dirty vulva? Does anyone care if I'm allergic to that lovely-smelling lavender in a body wash that is supposed to also make my vulva smell like a spring-time breeze? *They don't.*

There's no third-party certifying organization that verifies any claim or indicates that testing was done. In fact, the American College of Obstetricians and Gynecologists (ACOG) flat out states that "deodorants, perfumes, dyes, shampoos" are vulvar irritants[56] and they do not recommend "sprays, deodorants and douches" to address odor. These very products can actually be creating odor caused by conditions resulting from product use.[57] That doesn't sound very "clean," "fresh," or "sexy" to me. And it certainly doesn't sound good for my health. Gynecologists across the board tell women to steer clear of any fragranced intimate care product, yet manufacturers seem to enjoy coming up with new scents with names worthy of an eyeroll. Some doctors advise avoiding this product category entirely.[58]

There's a huge difference between a market study that generates marketing messaging like "Gynecologist Tested" and a scientific study.[59] Most intimate care products are in fact "regulated" (or woefully under-regulated) by the FDA as cosmetics rather than as drugs. Companies can use virtually any raw material in a finished product without FDA pre-market safety testing or review.[60] Companies are also not required to test the impact of an intimate care product on the vaginal microbiome. That's right: Products made to be used in and around the vagina are not required to pass any sort of FDA safety standard on how they may impact the very area of the body they are designed to be used on.[61]

Even the Summer's Eve mini-site, headlined to healthcare professionals and geared specifically to encourage providers to recommend the product to their patients, completely avoids mentioning "health." Instead, we see the language of clean, freshness, and self-care.[62] Removing or replacing smell does not improve health. I am fully convinced that any corporate lawyer knows this and has provided sound advice on just what manufacturers can claim these products do for the body.

Where's the Harm?

I get it. I, too, want to be "fresh." I keep the "house" tidy. I certainly want to take care of my health. I would even argue that there are some pretty hip companies new to the intimate care scene that are reportedly working hard to overcome decades of poor product offerings, toxic marketing, and more. Companies with potentially less harmful intimate care products (although I'm not convinced that any of these products are needed) compete with an industry that has long benefitted from the fact that women got the message that their vaginas are dirty and in need of a fix, a fragrance fix.

Putting aside the general lack of health benefits, where is the harm in these products?

As touched on above, intimate care products are regulated by the FDA as cosmetics. At the end of 2022, President Biden signed into law the Omnibus Spending bill, which included the Modernization of Cosmetics Regulation Act of 2022 (MoCRA). *MoCRA is the first time that federal cosmetics law has been updated in over 80 years.* The law that had been regulating cosmetics in the US since 1938 was only three pages long, and essentially allowed the industry to self-regulate. That's over eight decades of poor regulatory damage MoCRA is now attempting to address. MoCRA does provide important steps forward in the regulation of cosmetics and the future of ingredient safety, particularly regarding the disclosure of ingredients in professional salon products. It also gives the FDA authority to issue product recalls, and it requires mandatory adverse health events reporting by companies to the FDA. But the law continues to fall short in banning known harmful ingredients and does little to address overall product safety. There continues to be a lack of safety substantiation provisions or standards that cosmetics and personal care products need to meet before these products can go on the shelves and on our bodies. MoCRA codifies an undefined definition of "safe" that ignores long-term health impacts.

And it continues to give fragrance ingredients a free pass in almost every regard, with one significant exception; a short list of fragrance allergens will now be required to be listed on the ingredient label, although MoCRA does not require all fragrance allergens to be disclosed on product labels.

Companies will still be legally allowed to hide many fragrance ingredients (i.e., the chemicals used to make sure your vulva smells like a "Delicate Breeze"[63])—even if those ingredients are associated with reproductive harm, infertility, hormone disruption, cancer, and more. The fragrance industry can still govern its kingdom by its own rules. It has long shielded itself in secrecy and used its own definition of safety. Significantly, the vast majority of scientific studies on fragrance materials are generated by major fragrance manufacturers or the fragrance trade association's own laboratories.[64]

It turns out that there is a lot to be concerned about in terms of intimate care product ingredient safety. When I started working in communications in the environmental health sector, one of the first campaigns I worked on was called "Summer's Deceive,"[65] our organization's riff on the brand Summer's Eve. We called out toxic marketing language that was used to, as one advocate put it, "push products that make us feel like our bodies are dirty."[66] The campaign had a two-fold focus that spotlighted concerning toxic ingredients in the products. These included everything from formaldehyde releasers to a spermicide used in their wipes. The following is an abbreviated list of concerning chemicals that were found in Summer's Eve products. Reminder: These are products designed to be used on the vulva.

- **Octoxynol-9:** A potent contraceptive drug that effectively kills sperm.
- **Methylparaben and propylparaben:** Exposure to parabens is associated with genital rashes. Studies have also linked parabens to fertility problems and endocrine disruption.
- **2-bromo-2-nitropropane-1,3-diol:** These are formaldehyde releasers; formaldehyde is a human carcinogen. Exposure to formaldehyde can also cause allergic reactions for those who are sensitized to it.
- **Ext. Violet 2, Red 33, and FD&C Yellow #5:** Ext. Violet 2 and Red 33 are not to be used in products that come into contact with mucous membranes, and Yellow #5 requires a specific safety warning regarding allergic reactions when used in vaginal drugs.
- **Neutresse®:** A trademarked "odor-control" technology. Ingredients and potential impacts of ingredients are kept secret from the public.
- **Fragrance:** At the time of this campaign, fragrance was used in *all* Summer's Eve products, but labels did not provide fragrance ingredient information.[67]

I am happy to report that since the Summer's Deceive campaign was launched, Summer's Eve has now removed a number of these chemicals of concern, although others remain and new ones have been introduced. Those changes didn't come without years of work (including multiple letters signed by numerous health officials and organizations, over 15,000 petition signatures, a rally outside their corporate headquarters, and a lot of public pressure)—and these changes certainly did not come from any regulations or required safety measures. Summer's Eve didn't even start offering a fragrance-free option until 2019; and I might add that even their so-called "fragrance-free" products are filled with fragrance ingredients.[68]

What we *know* about certain ingredients in these products is cause for alarm. There's still a lot we *don't know,* particularly regarding chemicals used to make up fragrances. A single scent can be made up of dozens to hundreds of different chemicals. This isn't isolated to intimate care products. There is no federal law that requires manufacturers to disclose the chemicals used in fragrances, whether they are used in cleaning products, cosmetics, baby products, douches, professional salon products, menstrual products—you name it. While some companies are voluntarily disclosing their fragrance ingredients, the overwhelming majority use the catch-all term "fragrance" to represent any number of actual ingredients.

Take a minute to grab your bottle of shampoo (or wipes, or dish soap, or detergent, or lotion, etc.). Chances are you'll find in the list of ingredients "fragrance" or "perfume," or sometimes they'll get extra fancy and say something like "essential oils" or "natural fragrance."

In a world where corporate accountability is up to the corporation, fragrance-free products can be filled with fragrance ingredients. "Unscented" products often contain "fragrance" used as a masking agent to neutralize smells. Genital wipes can contain a spermicide without including any sort of warning, explanation, or apology to women who are dealing with infertility. While racking their brains for answers and blaming their bodies, women rightfully expect products sold to them to be safe and *not* to contain chemicals designed to reduce fertility.

These products also should not cause bacterial vaginosis. There is growing evidence to suggest that intimate care products are linked to infection by inhibiting the growth of healthy bacteria in the vagina (namely lactobacilli).[69] Disruptions of good bacteria in the vagina can lead to significant health problems, including bacterial vaginosis, yeast infections, unpleasant odor, increased risk of sexually transmitted diseases, fertility concerns, and possibly even cancer.[70,71,72,73] What's worse, many people often turn to these products to self-treat symptoms linked to infection, when in fact they could be exacerbating the infection. A 2019 snapshot survey of over 1,500 women in Boston found that more than one-third reported that they were *currently* experiencing one or more moderate to severe symptoms such as vulvar or vaginal itching, burning, discharge, dryness, and/or pain.[74] Over a lifetime, it is estimated that at *least 75% of women* in the US will experience episodes of vaginitis at some point.[75] How many of these symptoms were exacerbated by intimate care products?

As a reminder, many products are marketed as "gynecologist-tested." Yet a recent study (released by Women's Voices for the Earth, Black Women for Wellness, Apothercare, and CLIP Labs) that specifically tested several intimate care products to determine if they impacted the growth of lactobacilli found that some vaginal washes (including Vagisil Scentsitive Scents Daily Intimate Wash: Peach Blossom) significantly inhibited lactobacillus growth.[76] This Vagisil product claims it is pH balanced and "gynecologist-tested." I would hope that such testing would include impacts on the health of the vaginal microbiome, but when I see other test results showing inhibition of lactobacillus, I wonder exactly what sort of safety standards are being considered by the manufacturer. We still have no idea which specific chemical(s) found in this, and other intimate washes, are disrupting the vaginal microbiome. This also likely means, neither does Vagisil.

Marketing Targeting Black and Latina Women

Recent studies have linked douching or the use of "feminine" powder with higher levels of volatile organic compounds (VOCs) in the body, which is associated with cancers and neurological disorders as well as adverse effects in reproductive systems.[77] Another study in 2015 found that douching is linked to higher levels of phthalate chemicals, which are linked in turn to hormone disruption.[78] But those are just a few relatively recent studies. Studies published since the 1980s have reported health concerns linked to the use of vaginal "cleansing" products.[79] Regular douching has been associated in numerous studies with an increased risk of bacterial vaginosis.[80] Other studies link douching to cervical cancer, low birth weight, pre-term birth, HIV transmission, sexually transmitted diseases, ectopic pregnancy, chronic yeast infections, and infertility.[81] A 2021 study further links pelvic inflammatory disease (PID) to douching; PID can lead to various long-term reproductive issues.[82]

Yet, in the US, a 2002 study reported that one in five women between the ages of 15 and 44 still douched—and by 2017, the practice of douching had reduced to lower than 12% (*whew!*).[83] But the use of other intimate care products across the board is even higher, and it is growing. Cross-sectional studies in the US have reported that between 42 and 53% of women had used sprays, between 17 and 50% used vaginal wipes, between 23 and 46% used anti-itch products, and 2% used deodorant suppositories.[84] Data show that Black and Latina women report using intimate care products, like wipes, washes, powders, and sprays, at a greater rate than white women; and Black women report using douches over both white and Latina women, putting them at even greater risk for exposure.[85,86]

Why? It's complicated and complex, but also not bewildering—especially when examined through a historical perspective that links whiteness to cleanliness, as discussed earlier in this chapter. A research paper by Michelle Ferranti titled "An Odor of Racism: Vaginal Deodorants in African-American Beauty Culture and Advertising" documents the history of "pervasive olfactory discrimination" and its role in shaping ideas about cleanliness. Describing decades of racial bias evident in the strategic advertising of intimate products,[87] Ferranti specifically calls out the intimate care industry and outlines that no persons have been more impacted by marketing and messaging that creates, perpetuates, or manipulates the choices people make about caring for their bodies than Black women.

To give an example of how disproportionate harm can be so clearly linked to an industry's toxic targeting tactics, I'll talk specifics: Johnson & Johnson's (J&J) Baby Powder. To start, here are the ingredients in Johnson & Johnson's talc-based Baby Powder: Talc, fragrance. That's it.

For decades this product has been advertised not only as a must-have for babies but also for women to feel and *smell* baby fresh, baby soft. But as documents show, sometime in the late 1950s, J&J became aware that the talc used in Johnson's Baby Powder sometimes contained asbestos, known to cause health issues including cancers. Instead of warning the public about possible health risks, J&J instead doubled down on aggressively marketing its talc-based baby powder to women of color, distributing free samples in Black churches and advertising on Spanish-language radio. An internal J&J memo from 1992 acknowledged the potential links to cancer while simultaneously recommending increased marketing to African-American, "overweight," and Hispanic women. By 2006, J&J's own marketing analysis noted that 60% of Black women were using baby powder by this time, compared with 30% for the overall population.[88]

Fast forward to 2016 and J&J was facing over 1,000 lawsuits (and a $72 million settlement) for failing to warn users of its talcum-based products despite being aware of potential cancer risks.[89] Finally, in 2020, Johnson & Johnson announced that they would stop selling their talc-based baby powder in the US and Canada. They claimed this was due to a decline in demand.[90] J&J continued to sell remaining stock in the US and Canada. Despite ongoing concerns about this product's association with ovarian cancer and billion-dollar lawsuits and settlements, J&J also made it clear that they intended to continue selling this product globally, particularly in regions populated by Black and Brown communities. Following widespread public protest, J&J eventually announced that it would cease sales of talc-based baby powder globally by 2023. Again, the company cited "consumer needs" as the reason for this decision,[91] side-stepping the fact that as of October 2022 J&J was facing roughly 40,000 lawsuits from women claiming that Johnson's iconic talc baby powder was contaminated with asbestos, which caused their mesothelioma or ovarian cancers. One lawsuit was filed by The National Council of Negro Women, which accused the company of "deceptive marketing to Black women," despite internal concerns that the product might be harmful.[92]

There is some good news for the future of talc and cosmetics; the newly passed Modernization of Cosmetics Regulation Act of 2022 (MoCRA) specifically requires the FDA to create a standardized testing method for detecting asbestos in talc-containing products. While J&J will no longer be selling their talc-based powder, there are still talc-based products on the market and having a uniform testing method will help shed light on the scope of asbestos contamination in talc products. It's a start.

Johnson & Johnson might have ceased the sales of talc-based baby powder after decades of concerns and growing evidence of asbestos contamination. Summer's Eve might have removed a spermicide from their wipes and washes. Nonetheless, the residual trauma, harm, shame, confusion, and anger caused by marketing and selling these products remains. In the meantime, corporations attempt to distract the public with flashy press releases, statements of "no wrongdoing," and hollow messages of dedication to community and public health. These attempts to shift attention away from toxic business practices and into buzz metrics for board members eventually become lost in the headlines—and history repeats itself.

Where's the Point?

Vulvas are not supposed to be odorless. In fact, vaginal odor is important to help signal changes in the body to inform us about a health problem. But that's not the message we're sold, and unfortunately that's not the one we're buying. Advertisements for intimate care products have shifted away from adult women strolling through fields of wildflowers or riding a horse on the beach (while a voiceover proclaims how important it is to douche) to happy teens expressing their girl-power by spraying Berry Bliss on their vulvas before cheerleading practice. The narrative that these products are necessary to cure the curse of having a smelly, dirty vagina remains the same. One study from 2008 looking into why women douche found that women were nearly three times more likely to douche if they were concerned about a "fishy" smell.[93] In a 2003 study, 26% noted that they douche to reduce vaginal odor.[94] A 2022 study trying to understand why women use these products, despite knowing potential health hazards, quoted one participant who explained: "Well, mostly just smell and not wanting to have a dirty vagina, because I guess I had heard about all these things that you are supposed to be doing, and I wasn't doing them, so I thought like is my vagina not clean?"[95] And a survey by Vagisil from 2019 noted that 65% of the women surveyed were concerned about "smell" as one of their primary questions about vaginal health.[96]

Personally, I didn't need all these studies to tell me that women and girls are concerned about how their genitals smell. Fourteen-year-old me could have shared her constant worry about sitting too close to her lab partner the week her mom didn't buy the scented menstrual pads she usually used. So she sprayed perfume on her pad, convinced that it was the only way to hide any stink and keep her period a secret.

These survey results around the concern about "smell" aren't surprising. Why would these products exist if there wasn't something wrong with the way vulvas smell? Right? Because the industry has decided to loop menstrual management products and intimate care products together, the inference that people smell bad during menstruation is top of mind not just to teenagers but to women in my age group who will soon stop menstruating. Why would these products exist if there wasn't something wrong with the way periods smell? Right? *Or is it just me? What's wrong with me? Am I supposed to fix, reduce, and control my odor? Do others feel this way? Well, they must. And they must be doing something about it, so I had better too.*

Industry identifies problems and then sells solutions to the problems it creates—problems that don't exist. (See scented tampons.) Myths have a way of being turned into facts by amplification and repetition. *Wash, rinse, repeat* and repeat and repeat until the same idea has been echoed enough that there absolutely must be truth behind the need to keep my vagina smelling like Peach Blossom.[97] After all, why would this narrative be so dominating—why would a $28 billion "women's intimate care" industry exist—if I didn't have to do something to address the way I smell?

Such myths are repeated until they are part of our inherited "understanding." Take bears (yes bears), for example. Living in a location where bears might venture into a camping ground, I have heard repeatedly the myth that bears will smell menstrual blood and attack the offending human. This is not true. But that doesn't change the fact that I have heard a version of this myth ever since Girl Scout camp in the 1980s. Fast-forward 40 years and pamphlets printed by the National Park Service are still trying to combat this myth (often, unfortunately, by repeating it in an attempt to refute it).

Vulvas can and do have odor that doesn't need to be masked by deodorants. And any additional smell due to menstruation is typically unnoticeable, although menses may have a metallic scent. Olfactory sensitivity also fluctuates with the menstrual cycle. So the fact that your body may smell different to you when you are on your period is also related to how your nose works at that time of the month—not necessarily to any major change in the odor your body is emitting that others would notice.[98] Regardless, bathing as usual, changing your tampon, pad, cup, period underwear, etc. when needed is all that's called for.

Bodily shame (influenced by many of these bodily myths) has long impacted the way healthcare providers, educators, and individuals address vaginal health. A 2006 study of women from 13 countries found that less than half were comfortable talking with healthcare providers about vaginal health issues.[99] A 2015 survey out of the UK by Ovarian Cancer Action found that 66% of 18- to

24-year-olds were too embarrassed to bring up vaginal health questions with their physicians,[100] while another study noted that the majority of post-menopausal women avoid talking about vaginal discomfort with their doctor.[101] And it has certainly impacted the way decision-makers address this issue.

Former Congresswoman Carolyn Maloney worked for over a decade to get Congress to address the safety of ingredients used in menstrual products and intimate care products via legislation. A version of her bill, The Robin Danielson Feminine Hygiene Product Safety Act (most recently titled Robin Danielson Menstrual Product and Intimate Care Product Safety Act[102]), was first introduced in 1997 and has been reintroduced 11 times since the end of 2022. The aims of this bill seem straightforward: To require a research program to focus on studying the health risks of fragrance ingredients, pesticides, phthalates, allergens, titanium dioxide, and other ingredients used in menstrual and intimate care products. That's it: To see whether ingredients used in these products are harming our health. Speaking of straightforward, a bill reintroduced by Congresswoman Grace Meng asks for manufacturers of menstrual products (e.g., tampons, pads, period underwear, cups, etc.) to disclose their ingredients. Currently there is no federal law that even requires this very *basic* information.

Let's also not forget that many tampons and menstrual pads are bleached white without any discernible rationale other than a visual aesthetic. Exposure to bleached cotton may come with its own health concerns. What does bleaching suggest regarding ideas about white symbolizing clean/purity? Apparently, even the products we use for menstruation aren't pure enough without being bleached white.

The fact is, even if we can overlook the harmful impacts of the body-shaming narrative these products provoke, there is cause for concern about exactly what these products might do to our health. The vagina is one of the most absorbent parts of the body; this route of exposure is unique. It is alarming that even in the limited studies that we do have on intimate care products and links to adverse health effects, it is often unclear what specific chemical or chemicals are linked to harm. This is made even more challenging by fragrance. Not only do companies get to keep fragrance chemicals a secret (even if those chemicals used to make their signature scents are flagged as toxic), they also use scents and odor as the driving force to sell these products. In addition to fragrance, virtually all ingredients used in these products are not required to be tested for their impact on the vaginal microbiome, or to pass any third-party safety standards. Instead, the industry gets to define what is safe. And when studies continue to link the use of these products to health risks from infertility to bacterial vaginosis, I have serious questions on just what exactly *is* the industry's definition of "safe."

I'll repeat, because it bears repeating: What we *do* know about these products is cause for concern, as is what we *don't* know. They are both under-researched and under-regulated. These added exposures, and the risks (even the potential risks) companies are putting on women's health, are completely unnecessary and boarding on outrageous, all preying on our vulnerability to be "clean" based on the mythical definition industry has perpetuated if not created.

Yes, It's Personal

Does this sound personal? It is. What could be more personal than the products we use in and on our bodies? These are products we bring into our homes, the products we breathe in; that touch our skin, that we spend money on to help take care of our homes, our bodies, our families.

Do you know what else is personal? When you used Johnson & Johnson's Talcum Powder on your babies because your mom did, and because you loved that sweet, familiar, baby smell. It felt personal when you learned about damning links between talcum powder and cancers, and when you learned that that Tide® detergent (the one that triggered an urge to snuggle into the gray hoodie of your classmate) contains the reproductive toxin lilial[103] (a chemical banned from products in the European Union because of its toxicity).

Yes, this is personal. It's personal when you learn of your youngest daughter's love affair with the body perfume "Being Frenshe"—that has a trademarked undisclosed "Scent Technology" called "MoodScience"—also comes with a warning label:

FLAMMABLE. AVOID SPRAYING IN EYES OR ON IRRITATED SKIN. KEEP OUT OF REACH OF CHILDREN AND PETS. FOR EXTERNAL USE ONLY. USE ONLY AS DIRECTED.[104]

She specifically picked this spray because she's aware that not all scented products are created equally, and this one in particular is badged and branded by Target as "Paraben Free," "Cruelty Free," and "Vegan." And this product is also labeled *"Clean,"* which Target defines as products "formulated without phthalates, propyl- & butyl-parabens, formaldehyde releasers, ethanolamines, musks, nonylphenol ethoxylates, glycol ethers, problematic siloxanes & perfluorinated substances (PFAS)."[105] Yet the manufacturer keeps its fragrance ingredients a secret. There's that word again: *Clean.* And it was personal when my daughter asked which product is best for douching.

. I could suggest that choosing a consumer product starts with product safety, but that's not really the core issue. How we decide to take care of our bodies should be up to each of us. It's personal, after all. Consumer selections are based on personal and family histories, social and cultural norms, and how we respond to clever marketing that often plays a major role in the patterns of our everyday lives. I don't know what's best for your body, what makes you feel good, what makes you happy. Neither do the household or personal care industries, and they have a lot, a lot, a lot of resources to help convince us otherwise. What I do know for certain is that the products we choose to use in and on our bodies and to use in our homes should never put our health at risk. There is nothing healthy about toxic chemicals. Period. And it's time we turn the *Tide* (pun intended) and remember that "clean" should be something that not only triggers happy memories but keeps our bodies, our planet, healthy too.

Notes

1 Walsh C. How Scent, Emotion, and Memory Are Intertwined—And Exploited. *Harvard Gazette*. Published February 27, 2020. https://news.harvard.edu/gazette/story/2020/02/how-scent-emotion-and-memory-are-intertwined-and-exploited/.

2 Kadohisa M. Effects of Odor on Emotion, with Implications. *Frontiers in Systems Neuroscience*. 2013; 7(66). doi:https://doi.org/10.3389/fnsys.2013.00066.

3 Fortune Business Insights. *Perfume Market Size, Share* | Global Industry Report, 2026. www.fortunebusinessinsights.com. Published February 2022. www.fortune-businessinsights.com/perfume-market-102273.

4 cosmeticsdesign-europe.com. Strength of Scent? Still "More Room" for Fragrance Innovation in Beauty, says Mintel. cosmeticsdesign-europe.com. www.cosmeticsde-sign-europe.com/Article/2021/10/19/Fragrance-innovation-in-beauty-and-personal-care-targeting-wellbeing-holds-growth-promise-says-Mintel.

5 Fragrance Matters—Fragrance Is the Crucial Factor in Cleaning & Air-care Products, Survey Shows—ECJ. www.europeancleaningjournal.com. Published July 2016. www.europeancleaningjournal.com/magazine/articles/latest-news/fragrance-matters-fragrance-is-the-crucial-factor-in-cleaning-and-aircare-products-survey-shows.

6 Marmo S. Nielsen trade panel data for past 52 weeks ending May 8, 2021 for United States retail sales of laundry, surface cleaning, and dishwashing consumer products [unpublished report]. Procter & Gamble. 2021.

7 Scheman A, Jacob S, Katta R, et al. Part 2 of a four-part series, Hair Products: Trends and Alternatives: Data from the American Contact Alternatives Group. *Journal of Clinical Aesthetics and Dermatology* 2011; 4(7): 42–46.

8 Scheman A, Jacob S, Katta R, et al. Part 4 of a four-part series, Miscellaneous Products: Trends and Alternatives in Deodorants, Antiperspirants, Sunblocks, Shaving Products, Powders, and Wipes: Data from the American Contact Alternatives Group. *Journal of Clinical Aesthetics and Dermatology*. 2011; 4(10): 35–39.

9 Zirwas MJ, Stechschulte SA. Moisturizer Allergy: Diagnosis and Management. *Journal of Clinical Aesthetics and Dermatology*. 2008; 1(4).

10 Berthold D. Tidy Whiteness: A Genealogy of Race, Purity, and Hygiene. *Ethics and the Environment*. 2010; 15(1): 1–26. doi.org/10.2979/ete.2010.15.1.1.

11 Zimring C. *Clean and White: A History of Environmental Racism in the United States*. New York University Press; 2016.

12 Douglas M. *Purity and Danger: An Analysis of Concepts of Pollution and Taboo*. Routledge; 2002.

13 Smith V. *Clean: A History of Personal Hygiene and Purity*. Oxford University Press; 2007.

14 Casteel C. [Review of the book *The Smell of Slavery: Olfactory Racism and the Atlantic World* by Andrew Kettler]. *Journal of Southern History*. 2021; 87(3): 519–520. doi:10.1353/soh.2021.0094.

15 Nudelman J, Engel C. *Right to Know: Exposing Toxic Fragrance Chemicals in Beauty, Personal Care and Cleaning Products;* Breast Cancer Prevention Partners.

September 2018. Accessed June 2023. www.bcpp.org/wp-content/uploads/2018/09/BCPP_Right-To-Know-Report_Secret-Toxic-Fragrance-Ingredients_9_26_2018.pdf.

16 Scranton A. *Beyond the Label: Health Impacts of Harmful Ingredients in Cleaning Products.* Women's Voices for the Earth. April 2021. womensvoices.org/wp-content/uploads/2021/04/Beyond-the-Label-Report.pdf.

17 Nudelman J, Engel C. *Right to Know: Exposing Toxic Fragrance Chemicals in Beauty, Personal Care and Cleaning Products.* Breast Cancer Prevention Partners. September 2018. Accessed June 2023. www.bcpp.org/wp-content/uploads/2018/09/BCPP_Right-To-Know-Report_Secret-Toxic-Fragrance-Ingredients_9_26_2018.pdf.

18 Scranton A. *Appendix C of Unpacking the Fragrance Industry: Policy Failures, the Trade Secret Myth and Public Health.* Women's Voices for the Earth. 2018; 9–12. Accessed May 2023. https://womensvoices.org/greenscreen-for-safer-chemicals-list-translator-scores-for-fragrance-chemicals/.

19 Scranton A. *Unpacking the Fragrance Industry: Policy Failures, the Trade Secret Myth and Public Health.* Women's Voices for the Earth; 2018. https://womensvoices.org/wp-content/uploads/2018/09/Fragrance_Report_Updates_2018.pdf.

20 Scranton A. *Unpacking the Fragrance Industry: Policy Failures, the Trade Secret Myth and Public Health.* Women's Voices for the Earth; 2018. https://womensvoices.org/wp-content/uploads/2018/09/Fragrance_Report_Updates_2018.pdf.

21 Scranton A. *Appendix C of Unpacking the Fragrance Industry: Policy Failures, the Trade Secret Myth and Public Health.* Women's Voices for the Earth. 2018; 9–12. Accessed May 2023. https://womensvoices.org/greenscreen-for-safer-chemicals-list-translator-scores-for-fragrance-chemicals/.

22 Brennan B. Top 10 Things Everyone Should Know About Women Consumers. *Forbes.* www.forbes.com/sites/bridgetbrennan/2015/01/21/top-10-things-everyone-should-know-about-women-consumers/. Published January 21, 2015.

23 O'Reilly L. Some Marketers Moving Away from Dated Gender Targeting, Study Shows. WSJ. Published January 28, 2019. www.wsj.com/articles/some-marketers-moving-away-from-dated-gender-targeting-study-shows-11548673201.

24 U.S. Bureau of Labor Statistics. American Time Use Survey Summary—2021 results. Bls.gov. Published 2022. www.bls.gov/news.release/atus.nr0.htm.

25 Wolfe J, Kandra J, Engdahl L, Shierholz H. Domestic Workers Chartbook: A Comprehensive Look at the Demographics, Wages, Benefits, and Poverty Rates of the Professionals Who Care for Our Family Members and Clean Our Homes. Economic Policy Institute. Published May 14, 2020. www.epi.org/publication/domestic-workers-chartbook-a-comprehensive-look-at-the-demographics-wages-benefits-and-poverty-rates-of-the-professionals-who-care-for-our-family-members-and-clean-our-homes/.

26 Speiser E, Pinto Zipp G, DeLuca DA, et al. Knowledge, Attitudes and Behaviors of Latinas in Cleaning Occupations in Northern New Jersey: A Cross-sectional Mixed Methods Study. *Journal of Occupational Medicine and Toxicology.* 2021; 16(1). doi:https://doi.org/10.1186/s12995-021-00343-x.

27 *Cleaning Products and Reproductive Harm [Fact Sheet].* Women's Voices for the Earth; 2021. https://womensvoices.org/beyondthelabel/cleaning-products-and-reproductive-harm/.

28 Hair Stylist Demographics and Statistics [2023]: Number of Hair Stylists in the US. www.zippia.com. Published January 29, 2021. Accessed June 5, 2023. www.zippia.com/hair-stylist-jobs/demographics/?src=sp-popout-pageload.

29 *Nail Files: A Study of Nail Salon Workers and Industry in the United States.* UCLA Labor Center, California Health Nail Salon Collaborative; 2018. Accessed March 13, 2021. www.labor.ucla.edu/wp-content/uploads/2018/11/NAILFILES_2019jan09_FINAL_5a.pdf.

30 *Beauty and Its Beast.* Women's Voices for the Earth; 2014. https://womensvoices.org/wp-content/uploads/2014/11/Beauty-and-Its-Beast.pdf.

31 Kolmar C. 24 Powerful Cosmetics Industry Statistics [2023]: What's Trending in the Beauty Business. Zippia. Published March 2, 2023. www.zippia.com/advice/cosmetics-industry-statistics/.

32 Kolmar C. 24 Powerful Cosmetics Industry Statistics [2023]: What's Trending in the Beauty Business. Zippia. Published March 2, 2023. www.zippia.com/advice/cosmetics-industry-statistics/.

33 Exposures Add Up—Survey Results. Environmental Working Group. Published 2004. www.ewg.org/news-insights/news/2004/12/exposures-add-survey-results.

34 Nielsen Insights Reveal Black Dollars Matter: The Sales Impact of Black Consumers [Press Release]. Beaman Incorporated. Published February 20, 2018. www.prweb.com/releases/2018/02/prweb15226601.htm.

35 Beauty is More than Skin Deep for Asian-Americans. Nielsen. Published June 2015. www.nielsen.com/insights/2015/beauty-is-more-than-skin-deep-for-asian-americans/.

36 Helm JS, Nishioka M, Brody JG, Rudel RA, Dodson RE. Measurement of Endocrine Disrupting and Asthma-associated Chemicals in Hair Products Used by Black Women. *Environmental Research.* 2018; 165: 448–458. doi:https://doi.org/10.1016/j.envres.2018.03.030.

37 Dodson RE, Cardona B, Zota AR, Robinson Flint J, Navarro S, Shamasunder B. Personal Care Product Use among Diverse Women in California: Taking Stock Study. *Journal of Exposure Science & Environmental Epidemiology.* 2021; 31(3): 487–502. doi:https://doi.org/10.1038/s41370-021-00327-3.

38 Ding N, Batterman S, Park SK. Exposure to Volatile Organic Compounds and Use of Feminine Hygiene Products Among Reproductive-aged Women in the United States. *Journal of Women's Health.* 2020; 29(1): 65–73. doi:https://doi.org/10.1089/jwh.2019.7785.

39 Branch F, Woodruff TJ, Mitro SD, Zota AR. Vaginal Douching and Racial/Ethnic Disparities in Phthalates Exposures among Reproductive-aged Women: National Health and Nutrition Examination Survey 2001–2004. *Environmental Health.* 2015; 14(1): 57. doi:https://doi.org/10.1186/s12940-015-0043-6.

40 Berthold. Tidy Whiteness: A Genealogy of Race, Purity, and Hygiene. *Ethics and the Environment.* 2010; 15(1): 1–26. doi:https://doi.org/10.2979/ete.2010.15.1.1.

41 Women Intimate Care Market (Product Type: Intimate Wash, Liners, Oils, Masks, Moisturizers & Creams, Hair Removal, Powder, Wipes, Gels, Foams, Exfoliants, Mousse, Mists, Sprays, and Others)—Global Industry Analysis, Size, Share, Growth, Trends, and Forecast, 2022–2031. Transparency Market Research. 2022. www.transparencymarketresearch.com/women-intimate-care-market.html.

42 Intimate Wash Market by Distribution Channel and Geography—Forecast and Analysis 2022–2026. Technavio. Published 2022. Accessed March 5, 2023. www.technavio.com/report/intimate-wash-market-industry-analysis.

43 Feminine Wipes Market Size, Share & Trends Analysis Report by Distribution Channel (Hypermarkets & Supermarkets, Convenience Stores, Pharmacies & Drugstores, Online), By Region, and Segment Forecasts, 2020–2027. Grand View Research. Published 2019. www.grandviewresearch.com/industry-analysis/feminine-wipes-market.

44 OMV! by Vagisil TV Spot, "Oh-So-Fresh." www.ispot.tv. Published May 17, 2021. Accessed May 5, 2023. www.ispot.tv/ad/OGDh/omv-by-vagisil-oh-so-fresh.
   Following the launch of Vagisil's OMV! product the backlash was swift, as reported in *The New York Times* in 2021 (Blum D. When Vagisil Targeted Teens, the Backlash Was Swift. *The New York Times.* Published February 18, 2021. www.nytimes.com/2021/02/18/well/vagisil-omv-teens.html). Today, Vagisil has pulled this

product from the company website (url's like vagisil.com/omv are redirected to the landing page), but as of 2024, this line of products is still sold on Amazon, Walmart, and eBay.

45 Summer's Eve. Spa Luxury Daily Wash [Products]. summerseve.com. Accessed March 12, 2023. www.summerseve.com/feminine-hygiene-products/vaginal-wash/spa-luxurious-daily-wash.

46 Summer's Eve. Active™ Daily Performance Wash [Products]. summerseve.com. Accessed March 12, 2023. www.summerseve.com/feminine-hygiene-products/vaginal-wash/active-cleansing-wash.

47 CheapLubes. Coochy Body Oil Mist Botanical Blast 4 oz (118 ml) [Products]. CheapLubes.com. Accessed March 12, 2023. www.cheaplubes.com/collections/body-shaving-creams/products/coochy-body-oil-mist-botanical-blast-4-oz-118-ml.

48 Summer's Eve. Date Night Alluring Evening™ Daily Refreshing Individual Cloths [Products]. summerseve.com. Accessed March 12, 2023. www.summerseve.com/feminine-hygiene-products/date-night/date-night-cleansing-cloth.

49 Summer's Eve. Our Story. summerseve.com. Accessed March 12, 2023. www.summerseve.com/who-we-are.

50 Vagisil Wipes TV Spot. Storefront. www.iSpot.tv. Published January 29, 2013. Accessed March 12, 2023. www.ispot.tv/ad/7d1X/vagisil-wipes-storefront.

51 Summer's Eve—Hail to the "V" Commercial—extended cut [Video]. YolieOnline. YouTube.com. Published December 18, 2011. Accessed March 12, 2023. www.youtube.com/watch?v=e4Cs3Pp7mYg.

52 Lemisol Teen [Products]. thelemistore.com. Accessed March 12, 2023. https://thelemistore.com/en/products/lemisol-teen.

53 VeeFresh—VeeGentle Feminine Wash pH Balance for Women Wash with Apple Cider Vinegar [Products]. VeeFresh. Amazon.com. Accessed March 12, 2023. www.amazon.com/dp/B08Z4G9QY4/ref=sspa_dk_detail_4?psc=1&pd_rd_i=B08Z4G9QY4&pd_rd_w=xsfII&content-id=amzn1.sym.46bad5f6-1f0a-4167-9a8b-c8a82fa48a54&pf_rd_p=46bad5f6-1f0a-4167-9a8b-c8a82fa48a54&pf_rd_r=NAGJJ87539ERXNWEMDMR&pd_rd_wg=uJbf9&pd_rd_r=de159919-5331-43c7-870a-e08b934e255e&s=beauty&sp_csd=d2lkZ2V0TmFtZT1zcF9kZXRhaWww.

54 Johnson's Baby Powder Commercial 1989 [Video]. YouTube.com. Published May 18, 2014. Accessed March 20, 2023. www.youtube.com/watch?v=I-CrQ5kUfs8.

55 Johnsons Baby Powder Wedding Day Commercial. A Feeling You Never Outgrow (1986) [Video]. member berries. YouTube.com. Published February 3, 2017. Accessed March 12, 2023. www.youtube.com/watch?v=Y5-MCn8bXNI.

56 FAQ's Vulvodynia. American College of Obstetricians and Gynecologists. Published April 2017. Accessed March 2023. www.acog.org/womens-health/faqs/vulvodynia.

57 FAQ's Vulvovaginal Health. American College of Obstetricians and Gynecologists. Published January 2020. Accessed March 2023. www.acog.org/womens-health/faqs/vulvovaginal-health.

58 Gunter DJ. Merchants of Shame. *The Vajenda*. Published February 14, 2021. https://vajenda.substack.com/p/merchants-of-shame.

59 Stieg C. What it Really Means When a Product is "Gynecologist-Tested." www.refinery29.com. Published January 29, 2018. www.refinery29.com/en-us/what-does-gynecologist-tested-mean.

60 Product Testing of Cosmetics. U.S. Food & Drug Administration. Updated November 11, 2021. Accessed June 2023. www.fda.gov/cosmetics/cosmetics-science-research/product-testing-cosmetics#Who_s_responsible.

61 Product Testing of Cosmetics. U.S. Food & Drug Administration. Updated November 11, 2021. Accessed June 2023. www.fda.gov/cosmetics/cosmetics-science-research/product-testing-cosmetics#Who_s_responsible.

62 Summer's Eve Healthcare Professionals. Summer's Eve. summereve.com. Archived March 13, 2022. Accessed March 12, 2023. https://web.archive.org/web/20220313031415/https://www.summerseve.com/healthcare-professionals.

63 FDS Intimate Deodorant Spray, Delicate Breeze, 2 oz, Feminine Spray for All Day Freshness & Odor Protection; pH-Balanced, Talc-Free, Gynecologist-Tested [Products]. FDS. Amazon.com. Accessed March 20, 2023. www.amazon.com/FDS-Intimate-Deodorant-Freshness-Delicate/dp/B0163CSROY/ref=sr_1_2?keywords=FDS+intimate+freshness+delicate+breeze&qid=1667774598&sr=8-2.

64 Scranton A. *Unpacking the Fragrance Industry: Policy Failures, the Trade Secret Myth and Public Health.* Women's Voices for the Earth; 2018. https://womensvoices.org/wp-content/uploads/2018/09/Fragrance_Report_Updates_2018.pdf.

65 McConnell J. *10 Toxic Ingredients Gone from Summer's Eve, But Big Picture Problems Remain.* Women's Voices for the Earth. Published March 4, 2021. https://womensvoices.org/2021/03/04/because-of-you-summers-eve-removed-ten-toxic-ingredients/.

66 Tangirala S. We Shook Up Summer's Eve. Women's Voices for the Earth. Published August 16, 2018. https://womensvoices.org/2018/08/16/we-shook-up-summers-eve/.

67 Open Letter to Summer's Eve CEO. Women's Voices for the Earth. January 25, 2018. Accessed March 2023. https://womensvoices.org/wp-content/uploads/2018/01/WVE-Sign-On-Letter-to-Prestige-with-signatories-Jan-25-2018-FNL.pdf.

68 Conway B. *Summer's Eve "Fragrance-Free" Products are Full of Fragrance Ingredients?!* Women's Voices for the Earth. Published July 30, 2019. https://womensvoices.org/2019/07/30/summers-eve-fragrance-free-products-are-full-of-fragrance-ingredients/.

69 Fashemi B, Delaney ML, Onderdonk AB, Fichorova RN. Effects of Feminine Hygiene Products on the Vaginal Mucosal Biome. *Microbial Ecology in Health & Disease.* 2013; 24(0). doi:https://doi.org/10.3402/mehd.v24i0.19703.

70 Donders G, Van Calsteren K, Bellen G, et al. Predictive Value for Preterm Birth of Abnormal Vaginal Flora, Bacterial Vaginosis and Aerobic Vaginitis During the First Trimester of Pregnancy. *BJOG: An International Journal of Obstetrics & Gynaecology.* 2009; 116(10): 1315–1324. doi:https://doi.org/10.1111/j.1471-0528.2009.02237.x.

71 Atashili J, Poole C, Ndumbe PM, Adimora AA, Smith JS. Bacterial Vaginosis and HIV Acquisition: A Meta-analysis of Published Studies. *AIDS.* 2008; 22(12):1493–1501. doi:https://doi.org/10.1097/qad.0b013e3283021a37.

72 Wiesenfeld HC, Hillier SL, Krohn MA, Landers DV, Sweet RL. Bacterial Vaginosis is a Strong Predictor of Neisseria Gonorrhoeae and Chlamydia Trachomatis Infection. *Clinical Infectious Diseases.* 2003; 36(5): 663–668. doi:https://doi.org/10.1086/367658.

73 Mitra A, MacIntyre DA, Marchesi JR, Lee YS, Bennett PR, Kyrgiou M. The Vaginal Microbiota, Human Papillomavirus Infection and Cervical Intraepithelial Neoplasia: What Do We Know and Where Are We Going Next? *Microbiome.* 2016; 4(1). doi:https://doi.org/10.1186/s40168-016-0203-0.

74 Watson LJ, James KE, Hatoum Moeller IJ, Mitchell CM. Vulvovaginal Discomfort Is Common in Both Premenopausal and Postmenopausal Women. *Journal of Lower Genital Tract Disease.* Published online February 2019:1. doi:https://doi.org/10.1097/lgt.0000000000000460.

75 Lanis A, Talib HJ, Dodson N. Prepubertal and Adolescent Vulvovaginitis: What to Do When a Girl Reports Vaginal Discharge. *Pediatric Annals.* 2020; 49(4). doi:https://doi.org/10.3928/19382359-20200317-01.

76 Women's Voices for the Earth, Apothercare, Black Women for Wellness, CLIP Labs. *Intimate Care Product Testing: Impacts on Healthy Lactobacilli [Fact Sheet].* Women's Voices for the Earth; 2022. Accessed March 2023. https://womensvoices.org/product-testing-impacts-lactobacilli/.

77 Ding N, Batterman S, Park SK. Exposure to Volatile Organic Compounds and Use of Feminine Hygiene Products Among Reproductive-Aged Women in the United States. *Journal of Women's Health.* 2020; 29(1): 65–73. doi:https://doi.org/10.1089/jwh.2019.7785.

78 Branch F, Woodruff TJ, Mitro SD, Zota AR. Vaginal Douching and Racial/Ethnic Disparities in Phthalates Exposures Among Reproductive-Aged Women: National Health and Nutrition Examination Survey 2001–2004. *Environmental Health.* 2015; 14(1): 57. doi:https://doi.org/10.1186/s12940-015-0043-6.

79 Wong Ho Chow, Daling JR, Weiss NS, Moore DE, Soderstrom RM. Vaginal Douching as a Potential Risk Factor for Tubal Ectopic Pregnancy. 1985; 153(7): 727–729. PMID: 4073134. doi:https://doi.org/10.1016/0002-9378(85)90332-1.

80 BH Cottrell. An Updated Review of Evidence to Discourage Douching. *The American Journal of Maternal Child Nursing.* 2010; 35(2): 102–107.

81 Vaginal Douching and Adverse Health Outcomes, American Public Health Association (APHA). Policy # 20074. Published November 6, 2007.

82 Turpin R, Tuddenham S, He X, Klebanoff MA, Ghanem KG, Brotman RM. Bacterial Vaginosis and Behavioral Factors Associated with Incident Pelvic Inflammatory Disease in the Longitudinal Study of Vaginal Flora. *Journal of Infectious Diseases.* August 16, 2021; 224(12 Suppl 2): S137–S144. doi: 10.1093/infdis/jiab103.

83 Key Statistics from the National Survey of Family Growth, Douching, Vaginal. Center for Disease Control. National Center for Health Statics. Published 2022. Accessed March 2023. www.cdc.gov/nchs/nsfg/key_statistics/d-keystat.htm#douching.

84 Crann SE, Cunningham S, Albert A, Money DM, O'Doherty KC. Vaginal Health and Hygiene Practices and Product Use in Canada: A National Cross-sectional Survey. *BMC Women's Health.* 2018; 18(1): 52. doi:https://doi.org/10.1186/s12905-018-0543-y.

85 Branch F, Woodruff TJ, Mitro SD, Zota AR. Vaginal Douching and Racial/Ethnic Disparities in Phthalates Exposures among Reproductive-Aged Women: National Health and Nutrition Examination Survey, 2001–2004. *Environmental Health.* 2015; 14(1): 57. doi:https://doi.org/10.1186/s12940-015-0043-6.

86 Dodson RE, Cardona B, Zota AR, Robinson Flint J, Navarro S, Shamasunder B. Personal Care Product Use Among Diverse Women in California: Taking Stock Study. *Journal of Exposure Science & Environmental Epidemiology.* 2021; 31(3): 487–502. doi:https://doi.org/10.1038/s41370-021-00327-3.

87 Michelle Ferranti. An Odor of Racism: Vaginal Deodorants in African-American Beauty Culture and Advertising. *Advertising & Society Review.* 2011; 11(4). doi:https://doi.org/10.1353/asr.2011.0003.

88 Alcorn C. Advocacy Group Sues Johnson & Johnson Over Products Marketed to Black Women, Alleging Cancer Link. CNN Business. Published July 28, 2021. www.cnn.com/2021/07/28/business/johnson--johnson-talc-lawsuit-black-women.

89 Berfield S, Feeley J, Cronin Fisk M. Johnson & Johnson Has a Baby Powder Problem. *Bloomberg Businessweek.* Published March 31, 2016. www.bloomberg.com/features/2016-baby-powder-cancer-lawsuits/.

90 Johnson & Johnson Consumer Health Announces Discontinuation of Talc-based Johnson's Baby Powder in U.S. and Canada [Press Release]. Johnson & Johnson. Published May 19, 2020. www.jnj.com/our-company/johnson-johnson-consumer-health-announces-discontinuation-of-talc-based-johnsons-baby-powder-in-u-s-and-canada.

91 Johnson & Johnson Consumer Health to Transition Global Baby Powder Portfolio to Cornstarch [Press Release]. Johnson & Johnson. Published August 11, 2022. www.jnj.com/johnson-johnson-consumer-health-to-transition-global-baby-powder-portfolio-to-cornstarch.

92 Hsu T. Black Women's Group Sues Johnson & Johnson Over Talc Baby Powder. *The New York Times*. Published July 27, 2021. www.nytimes.com/2021/07/27/business/johnson-baby-powder-black-women.html.

93 Brotman RM, Klebanoff MA, Nansel T, et al. Why Do Women Douche? A Longitudinal Study with Two Analytic Approaches. *Annals of Epidemiology*. 2008; 18(1): 65–73. doi:https://doi.org/10.1016/j.annepidem.2007.05.015.

94 Ness RB, Hillier SL, Richter HE, et al. Why Women Douche and Why They May or May Not Stop. *Sexually Transmitted Diseases*. 2003; 30(1): 71–74. https://journals.lww.com/stdjournal/fulltext/2003/01000/why_women_douche_and_why_they_may_or_may_not_stop.14.aspx.

95 Jenkins A, O'Doherty KC. "It Was Always Just a Sacrifice I Was Willing to Make": Understanding Women's Use of Vaginal Cleansing Products in Spite of Adverse Health Effects. *SSM—Qualitative Research in Health*. 2022;2:100133. doi:https://doi.org/10.1016/j.ssmqr.2022.100133.

96 Survey: More than Two-Thirds of Millennial Women Have Turned Down Sex Because of Concerns About Vaginal Scent [Press Release]. Vagisil. Published August 21, 2019. Accessed March 2023. www.prnewswire.com/news-releases/survey-more-than-two-thirds-of-millennial-women-have-turned-down-sex-because-of-concerns-about-vaginal-scent-300904624.html.

I have a lot of questions on the questions Vagisil proposed in this study. Like did they ask if odor was a concern, or did they ask: What concerns do you have? Why is this important? There's a theory in communication that talks about the power and the predicament with "repeating the myth" in an attempt to actually bust it. Repetition of the myth helps solidify it by commanding the overall messaging and allows the myth to take control of the narrative and lingering message. One of my favorite examples of this is by Harvard Professor Alan Jenkins, who illustrates this theory perfectly in his attempt to convince his wife to agree to a brood of backyard chickens. Beyond the humor, Jenkins notes the sounding social science that myth busting "is worse than ineffective; it actually deepens audiences' belief in the lie. It reinforces your opponent's frame. And it exposes your opponent's frame. And it exposes the myth to new audiences who may not have heard it before." (Jenkins A. The Myth about Myth-Busting (and Chickens!). LinkedIn.com. Published December 30, 2017. www.linkedin.com/pulse/myth-myth-busting-chickens-alan-jenkins/.) There are tons of other chicken-less examples that are relevant to this discussion, but most of them are giant downers.

In relation to the Vagisil survey, depending on how this survey was conducted, I am very interested to learn how leading the questions were for the audience; if they presented the idea in the survey that women need to be concerned about vaginal odor, or if this is a topic that the respondents presented on their own. There is a huge difference between "Why do you use intimate care products?" and "Do you use intimate care products because you are concerned about odor?" Knowing the source, and that they used this information to promote a new line of products called the Vagisil Sensitive ScentsTM Collection, I have a hard time believing that they didn't feel it was important to bring "odor" into the conversation.

Vagisil, however, have no intention of busting the myth and rather build their brand with it. To quote their press release: "Today, Vagisil released findings from its Vagisil Scentsus, a survey of 1,000 women on a topic often taboo—vaginal scent." (Survey: More than Two-Thirds of Millennial Women Have Turned Down Sex Because of Concerns About Vaginal Scent [Press Release]. Vagisil. Published August 21, 2019. Accessed March 2023. www.prnewswire.com/news-releases/survey-more-than-two-thirds-of-millennial-women-have-turned-down-sex-because-of-concerns-about-vaginal-scent-300904624.html.) (Related note: Every time a corporation uses a pun an angel loses its wings.)

You caught me, I too am repeating the myth of you-know-what in my hopes to bust them. But if you've joined me this far, bear with me, and in the meantime if you need a mantra to keep focused, try "vaginas are self-cleaning."

97 Scentsitive Scents Peach Blossom [Products]. Vagisil.com. Accessed March 12, 2023. www.vagisil.com/scentsitive-scents-peach-blossom-daily-intimate-wash.html.

98 Bogdan MS, Slavic DO, Babovic SS, Zvezdin BS, Kolarov VP, Kljajic VL. Olfactory Perception and Different Decongestive Response of the Nasal Mucosa During Menstrual Cycle. *American Journal of Rhinal Allergy.* September, 2021; 35(5): 693–699. doi: 10.1177/1945892421990308.

99 Nappi RE, Liekens G, Brandenburg U. Attitudes, Perceptions and Knowledge About the Vagina: The International Vagina Dialogue Survey. *Contraception.* 2006; 73(5): 493–500. doi:https://doi.org/10.1016/j.contraception.2005.12.007.

100 Moss R. Fear of Saying "Vagina" is Putting Women at Risk of Late Cancer Diagnosis. HuffPost UK. Published August 17, 2015. Accessed April 2023. www.huffingtonpost.co.uk/2015/08/17/ovarian-cancer-late-diagnosis-women-embarrassed_n_7996982.html.

101 Reiter S. Barriers to Effective Treatment of Vaginal Atrophy with Local Estrogen Therapy. *International Journal of General Medicine.* 2013; 6:153–158. doi:https://doi.org/10.2147/IJGM.S43192.

102 Maloney C. *Robin Danielson Menstrual Product and Intimate Care Product Safety Act of 2022*; 2022. Congress.Gov. www.congress.gov/bill/117th-congress/house-bill/8724.

103 Tide Original Scent Liquid Laundry Detergent [Products]. SmartLabel.org. Accessed March 12, 2023. smartlabel.pg.com/00037000138822.html.

104 Being Frenshe Hair, Body & Linen Mist Body Spray with Essential Oils—Citrus Amber—5 fl oz [Product]. Being Frenshe. Target.com. Accessed March 12, 2023. www.target.com/p/being-frenshe-hair-body-38-linen-mist-body-spray-with-essential-oils-citrus-amber-5-fl-oz/-/A-85360332?ref=tgt_adv_XS000000&AFID=google_pla_df&fndsrc=tgtao&DFA=71700000012735304&CPNG=PLA_Beauty+Personal+Care+Shopping_Local|Beauty_Ecomm_Beauty&adgroup=SC_Health+Beauty&LID=700000001170770pgs.

105 Target Clean. Target.com. Accessed June 2023. www.target.com/c/target-clean/-/N-p4n12.

2

TOBACCO INDUSTRY CORPORATE MALFEASANCE AND WOMEN'S RIGHTS VIOLATIONS

Are Human Rights Mechanisms the Antidote?

Kelsey Romeo-Stuppy

For the last century, the tobacco industry has been the epitome of corporate malfeasance. For decades, the tobacco industry withheld important health information, targeted vulnerable groups, and even manipulated the public through bad science. Slowly, the world began to realize the harms of tobacco and the industry's role in furthering the tobacco epidemic. Globally, tobacco control policies have become more widespread and effective, in large part thanks to the "tobacco treaty," the World Health Organization's Framework Convention on Tobacco Control (the WHO FCTC). Tobacco corporations have now been found guilty of racketeering[1] and charged with manslaughter[2], and have been held financially responsible for some of their wrongdoing.[1] It is estimated that nearly 22 million future premature smoking-attributable deaths were averted as a result of strong implementation of demand-reduction measures adopted by countries between 2007 and 2014.[3] And in 2022, for the first time on record, global smoking rates dropped.[4]

Because of these positive steps, many believe that the tobacco epidemic is over. Unfortunately, tobacco corporations are quick to adapt and have changed tactics to target "up-and-coming markets," chief among them lower- and middle-income countries (LMICs) and women. As George Washington Hill, president of the American Tobacco Company (ATC) from 1925 to 1946, allegedly stated, targeting women "will be like opening a new gold mine right in our front yard."[5]

While, overall, smoking rates are decreasing, tobacco use among women is decreasing at a significantly lower rate than in men, and in some countries women are smoking more.[6] For example, in France between 1980 and 2012, despite a 6.3% decrease in smoking among men, there was a 75% increase in smoking among women.[7]

DOI: 10.4324/9781003472711-3

Today, 200 million of the world's one billion people who smoke are women and 2.15 million women die from tobacco use every year.[8] Over 71% of those women live in low- and middle-income countries,[8] where the burden of tobacco-related illness and death is heaviest.[9,10] In addition, approximately 700,000 women are exposed to second-hand smoke every year, and 53% of annual second-hand smoke-related deaths are women.[8]

Tobacco negatively impacts women's health in many different and serious ways. "Women who smoke have an increased risk for developing cancers of the oral cavity, pharynx, larynx (voice box), esophagus, pancreas, kidney, bladder and uterine cervix."[11] They also double their risk for developing coronary heart disease.[12] Smoking also negatively impacts a woman's reproductive health, particularly during pregnancy. Smoking during pregnancy causes premature birth, low birth weight, certain birth defects, and ectopic pregnancy in which the fertilized egg implants somewhere in the abdomen other than the womb. Smoking during pregnancy also causes complications with the placenta, including "placenta previa and placental abruption, conditions that jeopardize the life and health of both mother and child."[13]

Not only are the potential harms numerous, they are also getting more severe. While men's lung cancer risk doubled between 1959 and 2010, the risk among female smokers increased nearly ten-fold.[14] Today, more women die from lung cancer than from breast cancer.[15] So why exactly do women choose to buy and use such a harmful and deadly consumer product? It's certainly not an accident; it's a business plan.

Tobacco Advertising

The tobacco industry has been marketing to women in high-income countries like the United States (US), Great Britain and Spain since as early as the 1920s.[16] From the beginning, advertising campaigns in women's lifestyle magazines promoted cigarettes, using themes of independence, fashion, and thinness, such as "Reach for a Lucky instead of a sweet."[16] Magazine cigarette advertisements often featured famous models or movie stars.[17] Throughout the twentieth century and beyond, cigarettes and smoking were used as a symbol of glamor and women's independence.[16]

In the 1960s, Philip Morris began marketing its Virginia Slims cigarettes to women with an advertising strategy "showing canny insight into the importance of the emerging women's movement." The slogan "You've come a long way, Baby" later gave way to "It's a woman thing" in the mid-1990s, and more recently the "Find your voice" campaign featuring women of diverse racial and ethnic backgrounds. The underlying message of these campaigns has been that smoking is related to women's freedom, emancipation, and empowerment. According to the 2001 US Surgeon General's Report, "one of the most common advertisement themes in developed countries is that smoking is both a passport to and a symbol of the independence and success of the modern women."[17]

Tobacco companies extensively researched women's personal and social preferences related to smoking in order to create appealing packaging.[16] The advertising campaigns typically incorporated cigarette packs with stereotypically feminine themes, such as flowers, butterflies, and colors (e.g., pastel pink). "Slim or ultra-thin cigarettes were designed to reinforce the perception of smoking as a feminine, graceful, stylish activity that aligned with the idealized thin and glamourous images of women promoted in magazine ads."[16]

Women are more likely than men to smoke "light" cigarettes (63% versus 46%), often in the mistaken belief that they are healthier or safer.[18] In fact, "*light* smokers often engage in compensatory smoking, inhaling more deeply and more frequently to absorb the desired amount of nicotine."[18] Advertising is also used to reduce women's fear of the harmful health effects of smoking by utilizing positive, "healthy" imagery, such as "models engaged in exercise or pictures of white-capped mountains against a background of clear blue skies."[17]

More recently, women's desire for "safer" products suggests that it is a strong target market for novel products that tobacco companies market as "safer," such as heated tobacco products or e-cigarettes. "The gender-specific marketing for cigarette brands like Virginia Slims in the 1990s are replicated in the marketing for the new products IQOS, Blu, Glo or Vype."[8]

Unfortunately, it works. Collectively, these marketing strategies were effective at increasing cigarette sales and smoking rates among women. Studies have shown that tobacco marketing has a substantial influence over smokers and non-smokers. For instance, "one-third of youth experimentation occurs as a result of exposure to tobacco advertising, promotion, and sponsorship, and 78% of youth aged 13–15ʹreport regular exposure to tobacco marketing worldwide." This strongly contributes to turning youth-aged individuals into smokers.[19]

Regrettably, this is not all in the past. The Framework Convention on Tobacco Control (the "tobacco treaty") encourages countries to ban advertising, but one study found that only 18% of the world population is covered by the "highest level" of bans.[20] Even that high-level ban does not include common promotions, such as the retail display of tobacco products, on-pack branding, and, importantly, online promotions.[20] The tobacco industry has stayed current, finding a series of what seem like never-ending loopholes for its advertising tactics. In 2021, British US American Tobacco "invested GBP £1 billion in promoting its novel addictive products on TikTok where 60% of users are women."[8]

The industry also used the COVID-19 pandemic to its advantage. British American Tobacco promoted its product Glo in 2020, featuring women safe in quarantine using masks branded with the e-cigarette's name.[21] In addition, tobacco companies were found to have originated misinformation suggesting that nicotine protects against COVID-19, ignoring the evidence that smoking

worsens outcomes for those infected with COVID-19 as well as other data showing that vaping is associated with an increased risk for developing COVID-19.[21]

Tobacco companies sponsor women-related initiatives to garner business as
well. Every year, tobacco companies observe International Women's Day, but
a 2018 report revealed that Philip Morris International's public relations campaign on "Empowering Women" was rolled out in about 30 countries, largely
low-income and middle-income countries (LMICs), where a significant increase
in women's smoking has been observed.[8]

Tobacco in Low-Income and Middle-Income Countries

The tobacco-related burden of disease and death has shifted from high-income
countries to LMICs, with over 80% of the world's 1.3 billion tobacco users
now living in LMICs.[22] As women in LMICs become more empowered they
gain spending power, increased independence, and the societal acceptability of
smoking increases. The tobacco industry sees this progress as a harbinger of its
good fortune, as these conditions may facilitate increased smoking uptake among
women.[16]

The tobacco industry has already begun utilizing tactics in LMICs that
were effective in high-income countries.[16] For example, cigarette marketing
campaigns in India and the Philippines generally featured "women dressed in
fashionable Western-style clothing associating smoking with glamour, sophis-
tication, and independence."[16] Evidence suggests a pattern of international tobacco advertising that associates smoking with social advancement, similar to
that seen in the US.[17]

In addition, products targeted to women, such as slim cigarettes, lipstick in
packaging resembling cigarettes, and "light" or "mild" cigarettes are being advertised and sold in several LMICs.[16] For example, "the brand Yves Saint Lau-
rent introduced a new elegant package designed to appeal to women in Malaysia
and other Asian countries. National tobacco monopolies and companies, such
as those in Indonesia and Japan, began to copy this promotional targeting of
women."[12] Slim cigarettes that appear to be designed for women were associated with increased odds of experimental smoking among adolescents in China.
Studies in several countries found that teens and young women rated flavored
cigarette packs branded with stereotypically "feminine" colors as more appealing than flavored non-branded packs.[16]

The tobacco industry has continued to market "light" cigarettes in LMICs
as well. Despite "light" cigarettes being banned in some countries due to laws
prohibiting the use of misleading descriptors such and "light" and "mild," the
brand Mild Seven, designed to appeal to women, is still offered in some markets.
For example, a law in Thailand has a gap because the descriptor "mild" is only

banned in the "sub-branding," not the brand name. Japan Tobacco International has taken advantage of this loophole to introduce two additional variations of this brand.[23]

Smoking rates among women in LMICs tend to be lower than in higher-income countries.[16] However, in LMICs with the highest tobacco use, rates of smoking among women are more variable. For example, in 2018 fewer than 3% of women in Bangladesh, China, Egypt, Pakistan, India, Indonesia, Pakistan, and Thailand smoked. The smoking rates that year among women in Mexico (6.5%), the Philippines (7.0%), Brazil (9.5%), Ukraine (9.9%), Russia (15.7%), and Turkey (17.0%) were found to be considerably higher. In some of these countries, the smoking rates among women were similar to those found in higher-income countries like the US (16.7%).[16] Without intervention, the tobacco industry will continue to target women and girls as a large potential market for growth.

Marketing is a serious concern, but it is far from the only problem; the industry also influences policy-making and engages in aggressive litigation tactics that negatively impact women and girls, particularly women and girls in LMICs. For example, certain high-income countries permit tobacco corporations to manufacture cigarettes that have been determined to be unsafe for sale within their own (domestic) market and to export these inferior products to other, usually lower-income, countries. An investigative report on this practice concluded that "the cigarettes produced on Swiss soil and sold in Morocco are much stronger, more addictive and more toxic than those sold in Switzerland or France." These practices shift the burden of tobacco use to countries less capable of controlling marketing and sales and less able to deal with the health consequences of tobacco use.[22]

The hazards of targeted marketing exposure are multiplied in instances of intersectionality. Women who are part of other targeted groups such as the LGBT community, and, in some countries (like the US) are also people of color, are even more likely to be subject to marketing campaigns by the tobacco industry.[24] Tobacco is at the intersection of numerous human rights issues, and this amplifies its impact on many protected groups.

Other Women's Rights Concerns Perpetuated by the Tobacco Industry

Unfortunately, tobacco issues are more complex and more widespread than merely a woman smoking a cigarette. The tobacco industry creates myriad other issues that directly impact individual women and women's rights, including tobacco production, second-hand smoke, economic development, and environmental rights.

Tobacco Production

Tobacco production infringes the right to health and the right to education of women and girls. Women make up nearly 50% of the agriculture labor force in low-income countries[8] and in many countries around the world, including the US.[25,26] Tobacco companies use child labor to work tobacco fields, where they are exposed to nicotine, toxic pesticides, extreme heat, and other dangers.[25] Tobacco laborers are paid very little and often become ill due to the nature of the work. Exposure to nicotine in tobacco plants can cause acute nicotine poisoning, otherwise known as green tobacco sickness.[27] Human Rights Watch interviewed 26 children working on North Carolina tobacco farms in 2015, aged 16 to 17. Twenty-five of 26 children interviewed said they experienced sickness, pain, and discomfort from the work. While tobacco corporations state that they are opposed to child labor practices, the British American Tobacco and Japan Tobacco International firms have also gone on record to say that "light work in the fields that does not affect health or education is acceptable for 13–15-year-olds."[26]

There are many other nationally or regionally specific examples of unhealthy labor practices around tobacco. In India, bidis (hand-rolled) cigarettes account for 81% of tobacco smoking,[28] and 90% of bidi producers are women,[29] amounting to an estimated 10 million Indian women and children bidi rollers. These child workers are generally girls who drop out of school to help their mothers, and they often earn less than other bidi producers who make approximately $2 for a 12-hour workday.[30] Some of these bidis are produced by small, local producers, but corporations account for at least 39% of the market.[31] In addition to the infringement of their right to education, these girls and women inhale bidi dust, which is detrimental to their health.[7]

Economics

The economic implications of tobacco are multifaceted. First, tobacco is very expensive for the user. "The addictive nature of tobacco use crowds out other more productive household spending, such as purchasing food, education, housing, holidays and more."[8] Often that spending is from the households that can least afford it. World Bank studies of household disposable income estimate that approximately 10% of income in the poorest households containing at least one smoker is spent on tobacco.[32] Smoking also "increases the likelihood of falling into poverty, which fuels domestic violence, especially against women."[8]

Tobacco harms the economy at the macro level as well. The economic costs of tobacco use are substantial and include significant healthcare costs for treating the diseases caused by tobacco use as well as the lost human capital that results from tobacco-attributable morbidity and mortality.[33] In the US, the estimated annual income loss per capita (for people who smoke and non-smokers alike) was determined to be $1,100, as reported in *The Lancet* in 2022.[34]

The cumulative loss of income and unpaid household production was $864.5 billion (equivalent to 4.3% of US GDP in 2020).[34] The total global economic cost of smoking is estimated at around $US1.85 trillion, or around 1.8% of global GDP.[35] Smoking is expensive to both the government and citizens alike.

Second-hand Smoke

Globally, women are still the main victims of second-hand smoke, and more women than men are harmed or die from second-hand smoke (SHS).[8] In fact, "In women, the disease burden from secondhand smoke exposure is equal to or even exceeds that from firsthand tobacco use."[36] There are two main locations for second-hand smoke exposure: home and work.

Smoke-free air laws are viewed as a best practice for tobacco control, and have been implemented in many countries, although implementation and enforcement remain inconsistent.[33] Some workplaces that commonly employ women are not subject to those laws in many jurisdictions, such as private residences, bars, casinos, hotels, and restaurants.[37]

While exposure at work is a concern, the much greater concern is exposure to second-hand smoke at home. An analysis of second-hand smoke exposure in 14 LMICs determined that among reproductive-aged women, "Secondhand smoke exposure at home was common in all countries, ranging from 17.8% in Mexico to 72.3% in Vietnam."[38] By continuing to produce, market, and sell a highly addictive and deadly product, tobacco corporations are harming even non-smoking women around the world.

Environmental Issues

Every year the tobacco industry costs the world not only lives but also "600 million trees, 200,000 hectares of land, 22 billion tons of water and 84 million tons of carbon dioxide."[39] Tobacco products (and the companies who produce them) harm the environment throughout the entire lifecycle of the product, from growing tobacco plants all the way through managing post-consumer waste.

As the World Health Organization highlights, "The majority of tobacco is grown in LMICs, where water and farmland are often desperately needed to produce food for the region. Instead, they are being used to grow deadly tobacco plants, while more and more land is being cleared of forests."[40] The production, processing, and transporting of tobacco is equal to one-fifth of the carbon dioxide produced annually by the commercial airline industry, which contributes to global warming.[39]

Tobacco products end their lifecycle by contributing to litter and plastic pollution. As noted by the World Health Organization, "Tobacco products are the most littered item on the planet, containing over 7000 toxic chemicals, which leech into our environment when discarded. Roughly 4.5 trillion cigarette filters pollute our oceans, rivers, city sidewalks, parks, soil and beaches every year."[39] Cigarette filters contain microplastics and make up the second-highest form of plastic pollution worldwide.

All this pollution and the money and effort it requires to deal with it harms our planet and its inhabitants. The economic and environmental impacts create more prolonged droughts, reduced food production, and increasingly severe weather events that are disproportionately felt by women. The world's poorest countries are the most vulnerable; women make up the majority of the 1.5 billion people living on less than $1 per day.[41] Women aged 25 to 34 are 25% more likely than men to live in extreme poverty.[42] It is estimated that 80% of people displaced by climate change are women.[43]

Furthermore, according to the United Nations, climate change is:

> a "threat multiplier," meaning it escalates social, political and economic tensions in fragile and conflict-affected settings. As climate change drives conflict across the world, women and girls face increased vulnerabilities to all forms of gender-based violence, including conflict-related sexual violence, human trafficking, child marriage, and other forms of violence.[43]

Clearly, the climate impacts of tobacco corporations have deadly consequences.

International Mechanisms as a Tool to End the Tobacco Epidemic

Despite these alarming trends, there is some good news. First, women are highly motivated to quit smoking. "Approximately 70% of women smokers are interested in quitting and 55% make a quit attempt each year."[44] However, many governments choose not to make tobacco control a priority. That is when international legal and human rights mechanisms can be utilized to help protect the right to health of women around the world.

The human rights system is unique, because it is about the obligations of governments, not of private actors. The document "Guiding Principles on Business and Human Rights" summarizes the relationship between governments, corporations, and citizens in three words: protect, respect, and remedy.[45] A government is obligated to protect its citizens from the harms of tobacco and tobacco corporations, such as through the best practices laid out in the World Health Organization (WHO) Framework Convention on Tobacco Control (FCTC), discussed below. Corporations are obligated to respect those rights, yet they do not; the bulk of this chapter above illustrates how the tobacco industry willfully ignores human rights. If governments do not protect rights and corporations do not respect rights, citizens have remedies against the government.

The WHO FCTC provides evidence-based best practices on tobacco control. The FCTC is the first international treaty negotiated under the auspices of the WHO. It entered into force in 2005 and has since become "one of the most rapidly and widely embraced treaties in United Nations history."[46]

The WHO FCTC was developed in response to the globalization of the tobacco epidemic and is an evidence-based treaty that reaffirms the right of all people to the highest standard of health. The Convention represents a milestone for the promotion of public health and provides new legal dimensions for international health cooperation.[46]

The FCTC is essentially a blueprint for how countries can protect their citizens from tobacco and tobacco corporations.

First and foremost, every country can and should become a party to and accelerate the implementation of the FCTC. The FCTC has 182 parties, which amounts to a huge majority of countries; however, there are some notables missing, including the US.[47] The FCTC helps governments protect the health of their citizens through initiatives such as banning tobacco flavorings,[48] promoting tax policies that do not favor the tobacco industry,[49] and implementing standardized packaging.[50] All of these policies are important to protect women from the tobacco industry, specifically from targeted advertising.

In addition, governments should consider one article that is often overlooked: Article 2.1, which calls on governments to go beyond the measures specified in the treaty "in order to better protect human health."[51] Article 2.1 indicates that the FCTC is the floor, not the ceiling. Article 2.1 allows for governments that are party to the FCTC to move towards the ultimate goal of phasing out the commercial sale of cigarettes.

Human Rights Treaty Bodies

If governments fail to protect women from the harms perpetrated by the tobacco industry, the human rights system provides several potential remedies. There are multiple international human rights treaties on topics that are relevant to women and tobacco control. The International Convention on the Elimination of All Forms of Discrimination against Women has been ratified by 189 countries and is an international bill of rights for women.[52] Several articles in the Convention on the Elimination of All Forms of Discrimination against Women are pertinent. For example, the tobacco industry's misinformation, such as products like "light" cigarettes discussed above, has very frequently undermined Article 10(h) which protects access to educational information. Article 11(f) emphasizes the right to healthy working conditions, which is an important consideration in the discussion of second-hand smoke, a key issue for women.[52] Other international human rights treaties apply to women or specific populations of women as well, including the Convention on the Rights of the Child, the International Convention on the Elimination of All Forms of Racial Discrimination, and the International Covenant on Economic, Social, and Cultural Rights.

Several human rights bodies have already recognized the impact of tobacco. The Committee on Economic, Social and Cultural Rights, in its General Comment No. 14, asserted that the "failure to discourage production, marketing and consumption of tobacco" is a violation of the obligation to protect under Article 12.[53] Likewise, General Comment 15 of the Committee of the Rights of the Child noted that governments must implement and enforce the FCTC as part of their obligations under the Convention on the Rights of the Child.[54]

There are many opportunities to bring tobacco violations of women's rights to the attention of these and other treaty bodies. Government parties are obligated to report to each committee about the human rights situation in their countries regularly, usually approximately every five years. However, those reports seldom include tobacco. The reports are submitted to the committee for each treaty, which in turn makes recommendations back to the country that submitted the report. Advocates have the opportunity to submit reports and make oral statements and can urge each committee to consider tobacco control when implementing its mandate.[55] When a government has ratified a treaty, it is required that "its own domestic law and practice are consistent with what is required by the treaty."[56] In the US, for example, a ratified treaty has the same force as a federal law.[57] While General Comments and Concluding Observations from treaty bodies are not generally viewed as binding, they are persuasive.[58]

In 2010, several academic and civil society organizations submitted a parallel report to one produced by a Committee of the Convention on the Elimination of All Forms of Discrimination against Women.[59] In its concluding observations, the committee expressed concern about the negative impacts of tobacco on the women of Argentina, particularly about tobacco advertising directed at women. The committee went on to urge Argentina to ratify and implement the FCTC. This action was one of the first examples of a human rights committee making a specific recommendation to a government about tobacco control measures.[60]

Other International Mechanisms

The intersection of tobacco, women's rights, and other policy areas provide for interesting cross-pollination in the human rights arena. For example, as illustrated above, tobacco and tobacco corporations create a huge strain on the environment. Tobacco could and should be included in the negotiations around such agreements as the Paris Agreement, the Conference of the Parties for the UN Climate Change Conference, and even the new Global Treaty on Plastic Pollution, which is still a work in progress.

The United Nations Sustainable Development Goals (SDGs) and other frameworks that focus on development are another opportunity to include women's rights and tobacco. The SDGs are a "blueprint to achieve a better and more sustainable future for all" that has been agreed to by all UN Member States.[61] As the United Nations Development Program notes, the FCTC is an accelerator for sustainable development, and reducing tobacco use is critical to achieve every goal in the SDGs.[62] Tobacco control is integral to achieving the SDGs, and the SDGs are another tool to protect women's rights. All of these platforms provide opportunities to break down silos and work across subject areas to improve the status of multiple rights, including women's rights and the right to health.

Litigation

The tobacco industry has long used litigation as a tool to defeat public health measures. However, litigation works both ways, and another option for human rights victims of the industry to pursue remedy is through proactive litigation. Again, as human rights rely on the obligations of government, such cases would be brought against the government for failing to protect women from the tobacco industry. These cases could be brought in a human rights court, such as the European Court of Human Rights, or in a domestic court, utilizing human rights arguments. One recent example of the latter is a case from the US where several organizations sued the Food and Drug Administration (a government agency) for its inaction on menthol cigarettes.[63] Many of the arguments were based on human rights, especially on the Convention on the Elimination of All Forms of Racial Discrimination (CERD).[64] The lawsuit was successful, and the FDA is currently drafting a rule banning menthol in cigarettes.[65]

Of course, there are many other possible ways to pursue litigation against the industry. Some have been effectively utilized by the tobacco control movement. Examples of civil litigation in the US are the Master Settlement Agreement[66] and the Department of Justice RICO case.[67] Some legal tactics are cutting edge and just beginning to be utilized, like a case in The Netherlands that attempted to bring criminal charges of manslaughter against tobacco corporations and executives.[2] These measures are outside of the human rights system but may also be useful in protecting women from tobacco harms.

Conclusion

Tobacco products and the tobacco industry are a direct threat to women's rights, including the right to health, right to education, and right to a healthy environment. The tobacco industry knowingly infringes those rights, and governments often fail to stop it. The tactics employed by the tobacco industry are unfortunately extremely replicable by other corporations. For example, food corporations often utilize societal pressure to be thin to market so-called "healthier" or "diet" foods to women, similar to tobacco corporation campaigns suggesting "Reach for a Lucky instead of a sweet."[17] Marketing tobacco products to tobacco-naive women in countries with lax regulations sets an example for other corporations to shift marketing efforts for a variety of unhealthy products into unregulated territory.

The tobacco industry's lack of respect for human rights is egregious, and it has been extensively documented. After a "human rights audit" of Philip Morris, the Danish Institute for Human Rights came to the conclusion that "Tobacco is deeply harmful to human health, and there can be no doubt that the production and marketing of tobacco is irreconcilable with the human right to health."[68] While the tobacco industry stays in business, human rights, women's rights, will never be fully realized. Advocates for tobacco control have identified effective ways to halt this corporate malfeasance, and human rights mechanisms can be one effective tool.

Notes

1 Litigation Against Tobacco Companies Home. Civil Division. United States Department of Justice. December 2, 2014. Accessed June 7, 2023. www.justice.gov/civil/case-4.
2 Romeo-Stuppy K, Muller G. Update: Dutch Criminal Case Against Tobacco Industry. ASH > Action on Smoking & Health. February 15, 2019. Accessed June 7, 2023. https://ash.org/update-dutch-criminal-case2019/#:~:text=In%20September%20 2016%2C%20lawyer%20Benedicte,damage%20to%20health%20and%20fraud.
3 Chung-Hall J, Craig L, Gravely S, Sansone N, Fong GT. Impact of the WHO FCTC Over the First Decade: A Global Evidence Review Prepared for the Impact Assessment Expert Group. Tobacco Control. June 1, 2019. Accessed June 7, 2023. https://tobaccocontrol.bmj.com/content/28/Suppl_2/s119.
4 Drope J, Hamill S. Tobacco Atlas: Global Tobacco Users at 1.3 Billion; Smoking Among Young Teens Increases in 63 Countries. *Vital Strategies*. February 7, 2023. Accessed June 7, 2023. www.vitalstrategies.org/tobacco-atlas-global-tobacco-users-at-1-3-billion-smoking-among-young-teens-ages-13-15-increases-in-63-countries/.
5 Gil GF, Flor LS, Gakidou E. How Tobacco Advertising Woos Women: Think Global Health. Council on Foreign Relations. May 30, 2021. Accessed June 7, 2023. www.thinkglobalhealth.org/article/how-tobacco-advertising-woos-women.
6 Jafari A, Rajabi A, Gholian-Aval M, Peyman N, Mahdizadeh M, Tehrani H. National, Regional, and Global Prevalence of Cigarette Smoking Among Women/Females in the General Population: A Systematic Review and Meta-analysis. *Environmental Health and Preventive Medicine*. January 8, 2021. Accessed June 7, 2023. www.ncbi.nlm.nih.gov/pmc/articles/PMC7796590/.
7 Romeo-Stuppy K, Huber L, Lambert P, et al. Women, Tobacco, and Human Rights. *Tobacco Induced Diseases*. June 11, 2021. Accessed June 7, 2023. www.tobaccoinduceddiseases.org/Women-tobacco-and-human-rights,137473,0,2.html.
8 Women and the Tobacco Industry. STOP A Tobacco Industry Watchdog. April 6, 2021. Accessed June 7, 2023. https://exposetobacco.org/wp-content/uploads/Women-and-the-Tobacco-Industry-4.6.2021.pdf.

9 Sy D, Narian A. Issue Brief the Tobacco Industry and the Environment. *The Tobacco Industry and The Environment.* June 2021. Accessed June 7, 2023. https://exposetobacco.org/wp-content/uploads/TI-and-environment.pdf.

10 Tobacco. World Health Organization. May 24, 2022. Accessed June 8, 2023. www.who.int/news-room/fact-sheets/detail/tobacco.

11 Association AL. Women and Tobacco Use. American Lung Association. May 31, 2023. Accessed June 7, 2023. www.lung.org/quit-smoking/smoking-facts/impact-of-tobacco-use/women-and-tobacco-use#:~:text=Women%20who%20smoke%20may%20develop%20more%20severe%20COPD%20earlier%20in%20life.&text=Women%20who%20smoke%20also%20have,for%20developing%20coronary%20heart%20disease.

12 U.S Department of Health and Human Services. *Women and Smoking: A Report of the Surgeon General, 2001.* Accessed June 8, 2023. www.cdc.gov/mmwr/pdf/rr/rr5112.pdf.

13 Women and smoking—Centers for Disease Control and Prevention. *Women and Smoking.* 2014. Accessed June 7, 2023. https://www.ncbi.nlm.nih.gov/pmc/articles/PMC5928784/.

14 Lushniak BD. The Health Consequences of Smoking—50 Years of Progress A Report of the Surgeon General. 2014. Accessed June 7, 2023. www.ncbi.nlm.nih.gov/books/NBK179276/.

15 CDC WONDER Online Database, compiled from Compressed Mortality File 1999–2014 Series 20 No. 2T. Centers for Disease Control and Prevention, National Center for Health Statistics. 2016. Accessed June 9, 2023. www.cdc.gov/nchs/data_access/cmf.htm.

16 Czaplicki L, Welding K, Cohen J, Clegg Smith K. Feminine Appeals on Cigarette Packs Sold in 14 Countries. *Frontiers.* January 1, 1AD. Accessed June 7, 2023. www.ssph-journal.org/articles/10.3389/ijph.2021.1604027/full.

17 Surgeon General's Report (2001) highlights: Marketing Cigarettes to women. Centers for Disease Control and Prevention. July 27, 2015. Accessed June 7, 2023. https://pubmed.ncbi.nlm.nih.gov/20669521/.

18 Deadly in Pink. Campaign for Tobacco Free Kids. Accessed June 9, 2023. www.issuelab.org/resources/8943/8943.pdf.

19 Violations of the Right to Health Due to Inadequate Regulation of Tobacco in Argentina. United Nations Human Rights Council. November 2017. Accessed June 8, 2023. www.feim.org.ar/wp-content/uploads/2017/04/2017_epu_tabaco.pdf.

20 Freeman B, Watts C, Astuti PAS. Global Tobacco Advertising, Promotion and Sponsorship Regulation: What's Old, What's New and Where to Next? *Tobacco Control.* March 1, 2022. Accessed June 7, 2023. https://tobaccocontrol.bmj.com/content/31/2/216.

21 Big Tobacco is Exploiting COVID-19 to Market its Harmful Products. Campaign for Tobacco Free Kids. Accessed June 5, 2023. www.tobaccofreekids.org/media/2020/2020_05_covid-marketing.

22 Romeo-Stuppy K, Huber L, Toebes B, Yerger V, Senkubuge F. Tobacco Industry: A Barrier to Social Justice. *Tobacco Control.* March 1, 2022. Accessed June 7, 2023. https://tobaccocontrol.bmj.com/content/31/2/352#ref-16.

23 Japan Tobacco Inc and Japan Tobacco International. Tobacco Free Kids. April 2011. Accessed June 8, 2023. www.tobaccofreekids.org/assets/global/pdfs/en/Japan_Profile.pdf.

24 Tan ASL, Hanby EP, Sanders-Jackson A, Lee S, Viswanath K, Potter J. Inequities in Tobacco Advertising Exposure Among Young Adult Sexual, Racial and Ethnic Minorities: Examining Intersectionality of Sexual Orientation with Race and Ethnicity. *Tobacco Control.* January 1, 2021. Accessed June 7, 2023. https://tobaccocontrol.bmj.com/content/30/1/84.

25 Kasungu S. Child Labour Rampant in Tobacco Industry. *The Guardian*. June 25, 2018. Accessed June 7, 2023. www.theguardian.com/world/2018/jun/25/revealed-child-labor-rampant-in-tobacco-industry.

26 Wurth M. Teens of the Tobacco Fields. *Human Rights Watch*. March 28, 2023. Accessed June 7, 2023. www.hrw.org/report/2015/12/09/teens-tobacco-fields/child-labor-united-states-tobacco-farming.

27 Recommended Practices: Green Tobacco Sickness. Centers for Disease Control and Prevention. March 27, 2015. Accessed June 7, 2023. www.cdc.gov/niosh/docs/2015-104/default.html.

28 Parthasarathy K.S. Smoking Bidis Costs India Rs 80,000 Crore a Year: Study. *The Wire*. December 23, 2018. Accessed June 9, 2023. https://thewire.in/health/smoking-bidis-costs-india-rs-80000-crore-a-year-study.

29 Arora M, Datta P, Barman A, et al. The Indian Bidi Industry: Trends in Employment and Wage Differentials. *Front Public Health*. 2020; 8: 572638. Published October 7, 2020. doi:10.3389/fpubh.2020.572638. https://pubmed.ncbi.nlm.nih.gov/33117771/.

30 Aghi MB. Involvement of Women and Children in the Bidi Industry. Review paper presented at the WHO Framework Convention on Tobacco Control Conference; 2001; New Delhi.

31 Welding K, Iacobelli M, Saraf S, et al. The Market for Bidis, Smokeless Tobacco, and Cigarettes in India: Evidence From Semi-urban and Rural Areas in Five States. *International Journal of Public Health*. May 12, 2021. Accessed June 7, 2023. www.ncbi.nlm.nih.gov/pmc/articles/PMC8284861/.

32 Mentis AA. Social Determinants of Tobacco Use: Towards an Equity Lens Approach. *Tobacco Prevention & Cessation*. 2017; 3:7. Published March 2, 2017. doi:10.18332/tpc/68836.

33 Tobacco. World Health Organization. May 24, 2022. Accessed June 8, 2023. www.who.int/news-room/fact-sheets/detail/tobacco.

34 Nargis N, Hussain G, Asare S, et al. Economic Loss Attributable to Cigarette Smoking in the USA ... *The Lancet*. October 2022. Accessed June 7, 2023. www.thelancet.com/article/S2468-2667(22)00202-X/fulltext.

35 Vulovic V. Economic Costs of Tobacco Use. April 2019. Accessed June 7, 2023. https://tobacconomics.org/files/research/523/UIC_Economic-Costs-of-Tobacco-Use-Policy-Brief_v1.3.pdf.

36 Yang L, Wu H, Zhao M, Magnussen CG, Xi B. Prevalence and Trends in Tobacco Use, Secondhand Smoke Exposure at Home and Household Solid Fuel Use Among Women in 57 Low- and Middle-income Countries, 2000–2018. *Environment International*. February 15, 2022. Accessed June 7, 2023. www.sciencedirect.com/science/article/pii/S016041202200068X.

37 Johnson CY, Luckhaupt SE, Lawson CC. Inequities in Workplace Secondhand Smoke Exposure Among Nonsmoking Women of Reproductive Age. *American Journal of Public Health*. July 2015. Accessed June 7, 2023. www.ncbi.nlm.nih.gov/pmc/articles/PMC4455520/.

38 Caixeta RB, Khoury RN, Sinha DN, et al. Current Tobacco Use and Secondhand Smoke Exposure Among Women of Reproductive Age—14 Countries, 2008–2010. Centers for Disease Control and Prevention. November 2, 2012. Accessed June 7, 2023. www.cdc.gov/mmwr/preview/mmwrhtml/mm6143a4.htm.

39 WHO Raises Alarm on Tobacco Industry Environmental Impact. World Health Organization. May 31, 2022. Accessed June 8, 2023. www.who.int/news/item/31-05-2022-who-raises-alarm-on-tobacco-industry-environmental-impact#:~:text=Roughly%204.5%20trillion%20cigarette%20filters,build%2Dup%20of%20plastic%20pollution.

40 Tobacco: Poisoning Our Planet. World Health Organization. Published online May 29, 2022. Accessed June 8, 2023. www.who.int/publications/i/item/9789240051287.

41 The Feminization of Poverty. *UN Women.* Accessed June 9, 2023. www.un.org/womenwatch/daw/followup/session/presskit/fs1.htm.

42 Climate Change Exacerbates Violence Against Women and Girls. OHCHR. July 12, 2022. Accessed June 8, 2023. www.ohchr.org/en/stories/2022/07/climate-change-exacerbates-violence-against-women-and-girls.

43 Explainer: How Gender Inequality and Climate Change Are Interconnected. UN Women—Headquarters. February 28, 2022. Accessed June 8, 2023. www.un-women.org/en/news-stories/explainer/2022/02/explainer-how-gender-inequality-and-climate-change-are-interconnected.

44 A Lifetime of Damage—Campaign for Tobacco-Free Kids. Tobacco Free Kids. May 2021. Accessed June 8, 2023. www.tobaccofreekids.org/assets/content/press_office/2021/womens-report.pdf.

45 Guiding Principles of Business and Human Rights. OHCHR. June 16, 2011. Accessed June 8, 2023. www.ohchr.org/sites/default/files/Documents/Publications/GuidingPrinciplesBusinessHR_EN.pdf.

46 WHO Framework Convention on Tobacco Control Overview. World Health Organization. May 25, 2003. Accessed June 8, 2023. https://fctc.who.int/who-fctc/overview.

47 WHO Framework Convention on Tobacco Control—Parties. World Health Organization. March 3, 2021. Accessed June 8, 2023. https://fctc.who.int/who-fctc/overview/parties.

48 Erinoso O, Smith KC, Iacobelli M, Saraf S, Welding K, Cohen J. Global Review of Tobacco Product Flavour Policies—*Tobacco Control.* May 15, 2020. Accessed June 8, 2023. https://tobaccocontrol.bmj.com/content/tobaccocontrol/30/4/373.full.pdf.

49 Chaloupka FJ, Straif K, Leon ME. Working Group, International Agency for Research on Cancer. Effectiveness of Tax and Price Policies in Tobacco Control. *Tobacco Control.* 2011; 20(3): 235–238. doi:10.1136/tc.2010.039982.

50 Tobacco Plain Packaging: Global Status 2021 Update. World Health Organization. June 20, 2022. Accessed June 8, 2023. www.who.int/publications/i/item/9789240051607.

51 WHO Framework Convention on Tobacco Control Overview. Article 2.1. World Health Organization. May 25, 2003. Accessed June 8, 2023. https://fctc.who.int/who-fctc/overview.

52 UN General Assembly. Convention on the Elimination of All Forms of Discrimination against Women. December 18, 1979, A/RES/34/180. Accessed June 1, 2023. www.refworld.org/docid/3b00f2244.html.

53 CESCR General Comment No. 14: The Right to the Highest Attainable Standard of Health. Office of the Highest Commissioner for Human Rights. August 11, 2000. Accessed June 8, 2023. www.refworld.org/docid/4538838d0.html.

54 CRC General Comment No. 15 (2013) On the Right of the Child to the Enjoyment of the Highest Attainable Standard of Health (Art. 24). Convention on the Rights of the Child. April 17, 2013. Accessed June 8, 2023. www.refworld.org/docid/51ef9e134.html.

55 Submitted Reports—CEDAW: Sweden CEDAW. Action on Smoking and Health. Accessed June 9, 2023. https://ash.org/hrhub/reporting/.

56 Chapter 5: National Legislation and the Convention—Incorporating the Convention into Domestic Law. United Nations. Accessed June 9, 2023. www.un.org/development/desa/disabilities/resources/handbook-for-parliamentarians-on-the-convention-on-the-rights-of-persons-with-disabilities/chapter-five-national-legislation-and-the-convention.html.

57 U.S. Senate: About Treaties. March 3, 2021. Accessed June 8, 2023. www.senate. gov/about/powers-procedures/treaties.htm#:~:text=Treaties%20are%20binding% 20agreements%20between,supreme%20Law%20of%20the%20Land.

58 UN Human Rights Treaty Bodies. International Justice Resource Center. September 29, 2021. Accessed June 8, 2023. https://ijrcenter.org/un-treaty-bodies/.

59 Shadow Report to the Periodic Report by the Government of Argentina: Challenges in the Prevention and Reduction of Women's Tobacco Use in Argentina. O'Neill Institute. 2010. https://oneill.law.georgetown.edu/publications/shadow-report-to-the-periodic-report-by-the-government-of-argentina-challenges-in-the-prevention-and-reduction-of-womens-tobacco-use-in-argentina/.

60 Dresler C, Henry K, Loftus J, Lando H. Assessment of Short Reports Using a Human Rights-based Approach to Tobacco Control to the Committee on Economics, Cultural and Social Rights. *Tobacco Control*. 2018; 27(4): 385–389. doi:10.1136/ tobaccocontrol-2016-053517.

61 Sustainable Development Goals. United Nations. Accessed June 8, 2023. www.un.org/ sustainabledevelopment/sustainable-development-goals/.

62 The WHO Framework Convention on Tobacco Control. April 30, 2017. Accessed June 8, 2023. fctc.who.int/publications/m/item/the-who-framework-convention-on-tobacco-control-an-accelerator-for-sustainable-development.

63 Zhang D. Ngo Says Menthol Cigarette Ban Delay Hurts Black People. Law 360. June 17, 2020. Accessed June 8, 2023. www.law360.com/california/articles/1284099/ngo-says-menthol-cigarette-ban-delay-hurts-black-people-.

64 African American Tobacco Control Leadership Council et al v. United States Department of Health and Human Services et al. (Case 3:20-cv-04012 2020). Accessed June 8, 2023. www.bloomberglaw.com/public/desktop/document/ AfricanAmericanTobaccoControlLeadershipCounciletalvUnitedStatesDe.

65 FDA Commits to Evidence-based Actions Aimed at Saving Lives and Preventing Future Generations of Smokers. U.S. Food and Drug Administration. April 29, 2021. Accessed June 8, 2023. www.fda.gov/news-events/press-announcements/ fda-commits-evidence-based-actions-aimed-saving-lives-and-preventing-future-generations-smokers.

66 The Master Settlement Agreement and Attorneys General. National Association of Attorneys General. May 11, 2023. Accessed June 8, 2023. www.naag.org/our-work/ naag-center-for-tobacco-and-public-health/the-master-settlement-agreement/.

67 Litigation Against Tobacco Companies. Civil Division United States Department of Justice. December 2, 2014. Accessed June 8, 2023. www.justice.gov/civil/case-4.

68 Human Rights Assessment in Philip Morris International. The Danish Institute for Human Rights. May 4, 2017. Accessed June 8, 2023. www.humanrights.dk/news/ human-rights-assessment-philip-morris-international.

3

MOTHER'S LITTLE HELPERS AND OPIOIDS

Women, Addiction, and the Legacy of Arthur Sackler

Mary Hunter

Archeological evidence shows that human beings have long sought relief from pain and anxiety, and opium has been cultivated for medicinal purposes since at least 3400 BC.[1] A Swiss alchemist in the sixteenth century named Paracelsus prepared a substance he called laudanum from morphine, a product of the opium poppy, that he mixed with crushed pearls and other precious substances. The compound's name signified that laudanum was "something to be praised," and laudanum has since been used worldwide to relieve pain and anxiety. Even though men have certainly used laudanum, its use came to be associated with the female gender.[2]

Treating Pain and Anxiety in Early America

In the United States (US), laudanum bridged a gap between two medication classes: "patent" and "ethical." The word "patent" first appeared on products brought from England that were manufactured under grants from the Royal Family known as "Patents of Royal Favor."[3] Although few medicinal products sold in the US in the eighteenth, nineteenth, and early twentieth centuries were protected by US patents, some were trademarked, or branded, for marketing purposes. Drugs that could be purchased without a doctor's prescription came to be known as "patent medicines," and ads for patent medicines became a major source of revenue for American newspapers and magazines. Most of these ads featured women.[2]

Hundreds of branded medicines containing morphine competed for market share with similar formulations offered at much lower prices by pharmacists.[4] A second medication class, "ethical," signifies drugs that can be obtained only

DOI: 10.4324/9781003472711-4

after written prescriptions prepared by doctors are presented to pharmacists who prepare them for specific patients. Today, we call these prescription drugs. Like the word "patent," the word "ethical" didn't necessarily reflect the real world. Laudanum was readily available through either distribution channel.

Laudanum elixirs, or tinctures, were among the most common early patent (and ethical) medicines.[3,4] Consisting of morphine and alcohol in various ratios, patent laudanum elixirs usually included additional unidentified agents for added appeal. These trade-secret ingredients purportedly lent individual brands of laudanum unique properties, making one sound better for this, another brand ideal for that. During the Victorian era (Queen Victoria's reign was from 1837 to 1901), laudanum was cheaper than alcohol because it was taxed at a lower rate. It could be purchased in post offices, pubs, grocery stores, barber shops, tobacconists, pharmacies, and candy shops—it was completely unregulated. Claimed efficacy for laudanum ranged from relief of digestive issues to double vision, headaches to heart problems—it purported to help with just about anything, and it was advertised for use by both adults and children.

Women, Laudanum, and Opioids

The reason most advertisements for laudanum targeted women was probably because women were assumed to be prone to "hysteria."[5] This term had been used for anxiety in women ever since some Greek men, including Plato, blamed symptoms like panic attacks on the uterus. To the Greeks, mainly women suffered from anxiety, and sexual activity was suggested as a cure. During the Renaissance, some disruptive anxious women were called witches, and women with various psychological symptoms were tortured or burned at the stake. Doctors routinely recommended morphine for menstrual cramps, morning sickness, uterine and ovarian complications, and any type of nervous disorder a woman might exhibit. Over centuries, hysteria has become a rather loaded term. It is estimated that by the end of the nineteenth century over 60 percent of opium addicts were women.[4]

Early Opioid Regulation

The US Food and Drug Act of 1906 specified that certain drugs, including any containing alcohol or products of opium, had to be accurately labeled with all ingredients and quantities.[6] Additionally, state laws passed between 1895 and 1915 restricted the sale of all opiate-containing substances to patients with a doctor's prescription, thus limiting the availability of morphine as a patent medicine, but only in specific states.[4,6] Laudanum and other patent medicines continued to be legally sold in most states after 1906 if their contents were accurately labeled, yet sales of laudanum declined significantly after the Food and

Drug Act was passed. Thereafter, morphine was more likely to be dispensed by pharmacists and doctors, thereby lending it the aura of an "ethical" drug. An example of a contemporary ethical, or appropriate, use of morphine is treatment of neonatal abstinence syndrome resulting from maternal opioid dependence.[7]

Alternatives to Opioids for Treatment of Pain

Increasingly after 1906, the primary indications for laudanum were pain and anxiety (as opposed to laudanum being considered a cure-all). Fortunately, viable alternatives for treating pain became available. Acetylsalicylic acid had been synthesized in 1897 at the Bayer drug and dye firm in Germany and marketed as aspirin as early as 1899.[8] Availability of over-the-counter aspirin expanded quickly, and the use of laudanum for pain became relatively uncommon. Paracetamol, also known as acetaminophen, was also synthesized at Bayer in the late nineteenth century; however, this analgesic was not marketed in the US until 1950 due to concerns about potential adverse side effects that were later disproven. Because the inexpensive drugs aspirin and acetaminophen are useful for treating both fever and mild to moderate pain, and aspirin helps prevent cardiovascular disease, both drugs have been, and continue to be, widely used worldwide. Ibuprofen, introduced as a prescription medication in 1962, was the first of several additional non-steroidal anti-inflammatory drugs (NSAIDS) marketed to treat moderately severe pain. Over-the-counter NSAIDS are now inexpensive and widely available.

There are valid and important reasons why certain pain drugs are chosen for individual patients. For example, NSAIDs, including aspirin, should not be used by those with gastric ulcers or kidney disease, and acetaminophen should not be taken by people with compromised liver function. Aspirin, stronger NSAIDs, and acetaminophen do not produce drug dependence, and when they are used at high doses they can be as effective for treating pain as semi-synthetic opioids like hydrocodone, the active ingredient in Vicodin, and oxycodone, the active ingredient in OxyContin.[9]

Alternatives to Opioids for Treatment of Anxiety

When laudanum became somewhat difficult to obtain after 1906, anti-anxiety agents that could be substituted for laudanum were less available than were drugs for reducing pain. In fact, only one alternative medication class for treating anxiety was available.[10] The barbiturate drugs barbital and phenobarbital were synthesized at Bayer in Germany in 1902 and 1904, respectively. Marketed after 1902 as Luminol, phenobarbital was sold as a sedative, anxiolytic, and anti-seizure medication. Overdosing with phenobarbital is a serious risk, and successful treatment of an overdose is difficult. Even short-term use of phenobarbital and other barbiturate drugs produces rapid tolerance, and barbiturate withdrawal that is not managed carefully can be fatal. Sales of barbiturates rose dramatically during the Great Depression, partly because they were marketed as a safer alternative to opioids. (Sad fact: Luminol was used to euthanize children in Nazi Germany.) Only after 1951 was a doctor's prescription required to obtain barbiturates; despite this requirement, dependence became ever more common. In 1962, a committee set up by President Kennedy announced that there were approximately 250,000 Americans addicted to barbiturates (1962 was the same year Marilyn Monroe died from an overdose of barbiturates).[10]

No significant anti-anxiety pharmacology advances beyond barbiturates took place until 1955 when meprobamate, branded as Miltown, became the first psychotropic "blockbuster" drug in the US.[11] By 1957, one-third of all US prescriptions (yes, this is incredible) were written for meprobamate.[12] This was one of the first prescription drugs to be marketed to consumers, and it is worth noting that the manufacturer, Carter Products, was a former patent-medicine company. Carter employed flashy public relations stunts to draw media attention, such as commissioning a sculpture titled "Release from Anxiety" from Salvadore Dali for their exhibit at the annual American Medical Association convention. Their marketing firm was prompt in spreading the news when comedian Milton Berle announced that he used the drug and claimed to be changing his name to "Miltown" Berle.

The next drugs marketed to treat anxiety were benzodiazepines, starting with Hoffman La-Roche's Librium in 1960 followed shortly afterward by Valium. Marketing materials claimed that benzodiazepines were superior to barbiturates because they were "non-addicting." The 1965 Rolling Stones song "Mother's Little Helper" (penned by Mick Jagger and Keith Richards) was a commentary on middle-class Valium dependency.[13] Diazepam, marketed as Valium beginning in 1963, became the top-selling drug in the US by 1969. Other companies sold their own versions of *mother's little helpers*, with each new product advertised as superior to earlier benzodiazepines. The tactic of marketing, without evidence, newer benzodiazepines using claims stating they have lower addiction propensity, continues today.

From the turn of the century through the Great Depression to the 1960s, the pharmaceutical industry has steadily grown and become ever more powerful. Small companies that produced chemicals of all sorts made breakthrough discoveries with potential medical implications. Pharmaceutical industry growth was particularly stimulated by life-saving discoveries that were perceived as miraculous—work that led to two valuable classes of drugs. These drugs and associated classes were insulin and therapeutic hormones, penicillin and antibiotics. The development of these drugs clearly demonstrated that medicine could cure disease. Publicity surrounding the miraculous recoveries of people with diabetes and severe infections suggested that there was potentially a pill to cure anything. America in the middle of the twentieth century was a perfect place and time to sell drugs.

Arthur Sackler and His Marketing Innovations

Arthur Sackler was the eldest of three brothers from a hard-working immigrant family in Brooklyn.[14] As a young man he demonstrated remarkable intelligence, boundless ambition, excessive secretiveness, and a self-aggrandizing tendency when describing himself. As early as high school, Arthur began a marketing career that eventually put the Sackler family on a path to great wealth, high social standing, and notoriety. As editor of his school newspaper, Arthur persuaded the high school administration to let him sell advertising space and keep most of the income—something his predecessors had not thought of. Chesterfield Cigarettes was one of his main clients.

After Arthur completed medical school, trained as a psychiatrist, and completed a residency in a mental hospital, he encouraged his brothers Mortimer and Raymond to follow suit.[14] The three Sackler brothers' early experiences in the field of psychiatry stimulated an interest in psychoactive medications. Each of them spent only a brief time in clinical practice; they instead used their medical credentials to advance Sackler family business ambitions.

Arthur excelled in the New York advertising arena, and he continued to demonstrate that he knew how to structure a business contract to his advantage.[14] The marketing tactics he invented in the 1950s and 1960s presaged strategies still used today by the pharmaceutical industry. These include publishing fake doctor endorsements, bribing regulatory officials, designing and funding "scientific research" to support marketing claims, and lying about research findings. Such strategies were used by Arthur to market the benzodiazepines Librium and Valium for Hoffmann-La Roche. His tremendous success in increasing the sales of these medications (while "employed" by a firm in which he was a silent partner) was rewarded with generous payments linked directly to market growth. These were two of the most profitable drugs of the late twentieth century, and Arthur's share of Roche's profits funded the Sackler brothers' acquisition of drug-manufacturing firms and other investments. Arthur's success marketing *mother's little helpers* grubstaked the Sackler family's increasingly lavish livelihoods and allowed them to gain social standing by making showy donations of art and relics collected by Arthur (including an Egyptian temple) to museums in the US, England, France, Israel, and China.

In 1952, the Sacklers acquired the Purdue Frederick Company which sold Carter's Little Liver Pills and Senecot laxative, among other popular over-the-counter products.[14] In that constipation is a ubiquitous and often chronic condition worldwide, the company made money, but not big money. In 1966, the Sackler family purchased Napp Pharmaceuticals, a British firm that eventually contributed more significantly to the Sackler family's assets. Following the death of the (not-silent) partner in the advertising business that Arthur co-owned, Arthur and his brothers had a falling-out about a business arrangement the three brothers had made with that partner. In short, Arthur was cut out of overseas profits of Purdue Pharma and Napp Pharmaceuticals. Afterwards, Arthur and his brothers had little to do with one another on a personal level. Arthur, whose third wife was about the age of his daughter, became increasingly known to make promises he couldn't keep, including promises to his ex-wives. He secretly borrowed funds to continue making extravagant donations to museums, which kept the Sackler name prominent and sustained Arthur's reputation as a wealthy philanthropist. Arthur died from a heart attack in 1987, a few years before a major new pharmaceutical product, one that would help make the Sackler name infamous, was developed under the supervision of his brothers and their families.

Arthur's Brothers Bet on New Painkillers

The Sacklers had long sought another "blockbuster" drug—one that would make them richer than they already were.[14] After Richard Sackler (son of Raymond) took an interest in opioid pain relievers in the late 1980s, he organized a pain conference, the purpose of which was to spread the word that pain is not just a warning of a pathological condition. Rather, pain is a problem in and of itself, no matter what the cause, and failing to treat pain is unethical, unconscionable, immoral. Speakers Richard gathered at this conference outlined his argument that all kinds of pain—acute, chronic, post-operative, cancer-caused, whatever—. should be treated with stronger medication. Richard wanted to make the point that the medical establishment had been overly cautious about using opioids, that pain was shamefully undertreated, and that millions suffered needlessly.

In England, morphine and other opiates were, and still are, more commonly used than in the US, especially for cancer pain and at the end of life.[14] Napp Pharmaceuticals had introduced MS Contin, a strong, long-acting form of morphine in pill form, which was very profitable in England and other parts of Europe. Approval by the US Food and Drug Administration (FDA) was required to sell MS Contin in the US; however, time was running out on the patent. In order to sell as much MS Contin as possible before the name brand drug "ran off the patent cliff," the Sacklers neglected to apply for FDA approval before offering it for sale in the US.[15] After strings were pulled, legal action was not taken against them. Anticipating the MS Contin patent expiration and ever-increasing competition from drug companies that would be able to produce a generic version, Purdue's chemists worked diligently to add patentable features to MS Contin and to develop and patent another pain drug—one that only they could sell.

The new product, OxyContin, a long-acting, semi-synthetic opioid, was introduced in 1996 as a safe, non-addicting, oral pain reliever with reportedly few adverse effects.[14] Nevertheless, by 1999, Purdue executives had been repeatedly notified about their drug's addiction propensity and the resulting lethal consequences.[16] Speaking through their large and powerful legal team which included

Rudi Giuliani, Purdue denied any responsibility and asserted that all blame fell on "abusers" of the drug. Despite a growing death count, Purdue Pharma's marketing strategy continued to include broadening the indications for use and continued reassurance that, due to its long-acting formulation, OxyContin did not cause addiction. Purdue employed the term "pseudo-addiction" to indicate that a patient's withdrawal symptoms resulted solely from the fact that the prescribed dose was too low. Simply doubling the dose was suggested as the solution.

Purdue strove to expand the numbers of prescribers by sponsoring conferences, dinners, and trips, and generously rewarding the doctors who prescribed the most OxyContin and the drug reps who roped in the most doctors.[14] The company engineered the publication of continuing education materials and ghost-written medical journal articles that echoed marketing messages and contradicted existing science. These strategies mirrored tactics Arthur had developed for marketing Librium and Valium, tactics that had produced a benzodiazepine epidemic in the 1960s that is still raging. Although Arthur was no longer around in the 1990s, his innovative marketing strategies and the seed capital he provided enabled the Sackler family to create an opioid crisis that made an existing benzodiazepine epidemic look pale in comparison.

Substance Dependence and Women in the Twenty-first Century

Opioids and benzodiazepines are classes of psychotropic medications associated with an unprecedented drug epidemic, particularly in communities where OxyContin was marketed most aggressively by Purdue Pharma.[14] The use of opioids is often linked to the use of benzodiazepines, and women who are prescribed a drug in either class experience more severe health outcomes than do men. The over-prescription of opioids and benzodiazepines, especially to women, adversely impacts families and communities.

Opioids

Despite an overall decline in prescriptions between 2011 and 2022, opioids are still among the most widely used prescription medications. In 2016 alone, 11.7 billion opioid pills were prescribed, which was enough for every person in the US, even children, to have 36 pills each.[17] That year, 30 percent more women received opioid prescriptions than did men,[17] and the rate of opioid prescribing has continued to increase faster among women than among men, including seniors, who receive the largest share.[18,19,20,21] Deaths from overdose between 1990 and 2010 increased 265 percent among men and 400 percent among women.[22] Considering overdose deaths in women, those aged 45 to 54 comprise the largest group.

Women are more likely than men to seek medical treatment for a wide range of chronic conditions for which opioids are prescribed.[23] Treating chronic conditions with opioids is not recommended because tolerance develops within days, limiting their analgesic effectiveness. In women, lower doses of opioids result in dependence, and dependence occurs more quickly compared with men. Use of opioids as well as use of other medications associated with cognitive impairment can result in falls, and fall risk is particularly concerning in frail women.[21]

Women are offered treatment for opioid dependence less often than are men, and they are more likely to refuse it.[24] Reasons for resistance to treatment include stigma associated with drug use, concern about cost, financial or emotional dependence on another user, responsibility for childcare, fear of loss of employment, fear of loss of child custody, and safety concerns regarding mixed-gender treatment groups.[18,24] When they do enter treatment, more women than men exhibit behavioral and social impairment and are diagnosed with other psychological and medical illnesses. These factors not only contribute to substance dependence, they also often complicate treatment.

In the US, Approximately 56 million people every year receive prescriptions for opioids following surgery, and up to 24 percent of people taking opioid pain drugs of any type longer than three weeks become addicted.[17] Opioid-naive female surgical patients are at particularly high risk for persistent use.[25] Despite the recommendation of various medical organizations to treat post-surgical pain using alternatives, such as multimodal pain management (which can include acetaminophen, NSAIDS, and local anesthetics), the prescription of opioid medication is common. Opioid over-prescription not only leads to dependence, but unused medication is frequently passed on to family or friends, putting others at risk for dependence. Additionally, exposing surgical patients to opioids puts them at risk for side effects, such as nausea, constipation, and dizziness. While men and women are prescribed roughly similar amounts of opioids for pain following surgeries performed on both genders, 40 percent more women become persistent users than do men.[17] This difference is most pronounced in women aged 45 to 54, 12.8 percent of whom become dependent on opioids.

Opioid medications are often prescribed after obstetric and gynecologic surgeries. The most common obstetric surgery is cesarean section, which was performed at a rate of 32.1 percent of all deliveries in the US in 2021.[26] Only about one in 300 women become persistent opioid users following this surgery,[27] a statistic nonetheless concerning in that almost 1.2 million cesarean sections are performed each year.[26] Hysterectomy, the second most common surgery in women, has an even greater impact on the incidence of opioid use disorder. Over 500,000 hysterectomies are performed each year, and by age 60 more than one-third of all women have undergone this surgery.[28] Following hysterectomy, 7.5 percent of women become persistent users of opioids.[17]

Treatment of opioid dependence typically involves using an opioid agonist, such as buprenorphine or methadone, along with cognitive-behavioral therapy and treatment of comorbidities, such as pain or psychiatric illness.[24] Healthcare providers with a license to prescribe schedule III drugs can prescribe buprenorphine; however, methadone is usually provided in a licensed opioid treatment center or pharmacy. While some experts advocate tapering completely off the opioid agonist, there are those who argue for indefinite use of the drug to prevent relapse.

The market for buprenorphine is strong and growing, so there is cause for concern about conflict of interest. This is somewhat related to a broader discussion about whether addiction is a chronic relapsing brain disease (CRBD).[29] This disease model labels a person with CRBD a lifelong addict (i.e., a patient requiring ongoing treatment with no goal of recovery). Proponents of the concept argue that a diagnosis of CRBD destigmatizes dependence and facilitates access to treatment, while skeptics express concern that it marginalizes people, particularly those in certain social groups, and takes away their agency.

Benzodiazepines

Concurrent use of both opioids and benzodiazepines, as well as incidence rates of overdose deaths, have steadily increased since the early 2000s.[30] Approximately 70 percent of patients seeking medically assisted treatment of an opioid-use disorder also use benzodiazepines. The risk of overdose is significantly higher in individuals who use both classes of drugs, and almost one-third of overdose deaths involve both drug classes. Users often report that one reason they take benzodiazepines is to decrease the effects of opioid withdrawal.

Benzodiazepines are the most-prescribed drugs for anxiety and insomnia, particularly in populations of older adults.[31,32] Tolerance to, and dependence on, benzodiazepines can develop in two to four weeks. Dependence is concerning for many reasons, including increased risk for falls, potential inattention or slow reaction time while driving a car, and overall impaired decision-making. Benzodiazepines are used more often by women than by men, and users are more likely to be white and non-Hispanic.[31] Among women, benzodiazepines have been observed to be associated with cognitive decline and dementia, particularly at higher doses.[32] As noted earlier, benzodiazepines used concurrently with opioids significantly increase the risk for respiratory suppression and overdose.

Treatment of benzodiazepine dependence typically involves tapering the dose of the same benzodiazepine over a period of weeks or months.[31,32] Withdrawal symptoms can include tremor, sweating, insomnia, nausea and vomiting, hallucinations, agitation, anxiety, and seizures. Supervision of the tapering process is strongly advised, and hospitalization is sometimes necessary to achieve an appropriate gradual reduction in dose. The goal of treatment is to discontinue use of the drug.

Drug Diversion to Informal Markets

Diversion refers to the act of giving or selling prescription drugs to anyone who was not prescribed the medication. *Informal markets* are illegal markets—drugs for sale "on the street." This is where patients turn to obtain drugs they once thought of as medicines after they have been denied refills.[33] This phenomenon was effectively incorporated into the storyline of *Dopesick*, a Hulu mini-series about OxyContin over-promotion and the Sackler family. A large percentage of prescribed drugs including benzodiazepines, such as Librium, Valium, and countless other tranquilizers, as well as stimulants, codeine- and morphine-based drugs, and semi-synthetic opioids such as OxyContin, are diverted to informal markets.

Sometimes pills are crushed and inhaled or dissolved in a solvent and injected (rather than being swallowed) because these forms of delivery relieve withdrawal symptoms quickly.[14] In addition, using some drugs in this way can result in a feeling of euphoria, a "high." Purdue has patented pill formulations that require extra effort to crush and dissolve their products, yet these innovations constitute the company's only response to the widespread availability of OxyContin in the informal drug market. Moreover, Purdue's patents prevent other drug companies from using the same technologies to prevent abuse.

Countless people find themselves unable to obtain appropriate treatment for pain or anxiety, and in many instances appropriate treatment involves more than medication. Whether or not treatment requires the addition of physical therapy, cognitive behavior therapy, or another modality, appropriate treatment is not affordable or available to millions of individuals suffering from drug dependance.

By putting profits over human lives, Purdue Pharma and its competitors wreaked havoc on people from all segments of society; however, the opioid epidemic has not been experienced equally.[33] Because the justice system selectively criminalizes the use of drugs by the poor and people of color, people in these sectors have suffered higher incarceration rates, more poverty, greater morbidity and mortality, more drug dependence, and additional deleterious impacts on their families and communities.

Women, Incarceration, and the War on Drugs

The proportion of the jail and prison population made up of women—approximately 10 percent in the US—has grown since the opioid epidemic, and more than 60 percent of incarcerated women are confined for drug offenses.[34,35] Although the opioid crisis increased the number of white women in the criminal justice system, minority women are still incarcerated at higher rates—Native American women at six times, Black women at two times, and Latinas at a rate 20 percent higher than the incarceration rate of white women. These disparities exist despite the fact that drug use is similar across racial and ethnic groups.

Mothers of minor children, many sole caregivers prior to their incarceration, make up about 60 percent of state and federal women's prison populations.[34] Note that the majority of women charged with drug offences are held in county or city jails.[35] In most instances, because their incomes fall below the poverty line and they cannot afford bail, these women are held while awaiting trial. Approximately 60 percent of jailed women have not been convicted of a crime.

The children of incarcerated women are several times more likely to enter foster care, to drop out of school, and to eventually enter the criminal legal system compared with other children.[34] In many states, people with a drug conviction are ineligible for public assistance, and some social service systems require drug testing to process claims. Drug convictions are often handled in the child welfare system as equivalent to child abuse, whether a child is harmed or not, and children can be removed from the home for no other reason than alleged drug use.

Marketing OxyContin Outside the US to Maintain Corporate Profits

Because the use of opioid painkillers such as oxycodone (the active ingredient in OxyContin) has led to an epidemic of dependence, the medical establishment in the US has begun to emphasize the need to avoid over-prescribing these drugs, especially for chronic or post-surgical pain.[17] Consequently, numbers of new prescriptions for opioid medications have been lowered, numbers of pills prescribed for novice users have been reduced, and systematic de-prescribing of opioids using medically assisted treatment has been undertaken in both outpatient and inpatient settings.

Predictably, Purdue Pharma, taking a cue from the tobacco industry, has shifted its marketing efforts to other parts of the world through a sister company, MundiPharma.[36] One justification for marketing Oxycodone in other countries is the plausible supposition that cancer pain is truly undertreated in many parts of the world. Nevertheless, celebrities filmed in heavy chains (that represent their own pain) have appeared abroad in television and magazine ads for OxyContin, arguing that treating long-term chronic pain with synthetic opioids is morally necessary and medically appropriate. The advantage of appealing to a young audience is obvious. Cancer patients and old people are probably not users of OxyContin for very long, so why target them? Young and middle-aged people with chronic pain living in countries that have yet to experience the disastrous consequences of an opioid epidemic comprise a potentially huge market, one that Purdue-owned MundiPharma is determined to capture.

Notes

1 Cock-Starkey C. The Lure of Laudanum, the Victorians' Favorite Drug. www.mentalfloss.com/article/89268/lure-laudanum-victorians-favorite-drug.
2 Meyers T. *Journal of Victorian Culture*. December 18, 2020.
3 Institution S. Balm of America: Patent Medicine Collection 2023. https://americanhistory.si.edu/collections/object-groups/balm-of-america-patent-medicine-collection/history.
4 Trickey E. Inside the Story of America's 19th-Century Opiate Addiction. www.smithsonianmag.com/history/inside-story-americas-19th-century-opiate-addiction-180967673/.
5 Cohut M. The Controversy of "Female Hysteria". *Medical News Today*. 2020.
6 Musto DF. *The American Disease: Origins of Narcotic Control* (Third Edition). Oxford University Press; 1999.
7 Jansson LM, Patrick SW. Neonatal Abstinence Syndrome. *Pediatric Clinics of North America*. April 2019; 66(2): 353–367. doi:10.1016/j.pcl.2018.12.006.
8 Sneader W. *Drug Discovery: A History*. Wiley; 2005.
9 Frampton C, Quinlan J. Evidence for the Use of Non-steroidal Anti-inflammatory Drugs for Acute Pain in the Post Anaesthesia Care Unit. *Journal of Perioperative Practice*. December 2009; 19(12): 418–423. doi:10.1177/175045890901901201.
10 López-Muñoz F, Ucha-Udabe R, Alamo C. The History of Barbiturates a Century After Their Clinical Introduction. *Neuropsychiatric Disease Treatment*. December 2005; 1(4): 329–343.
11 Herzberg D. Blockbusters and Controlled Substances: Miltown, Quaalude, and Consumer Demand for Drugs in Postwar America. *Studies in History and Philosophy of Biological and Biomedical Science*. December 2011; 42(4): 415–426. doi:10.1016/j.shpsc.2011.05.005.
12 Tone A. *The Age of Anxiety: A History of America's Turbulent Affair with Tranquilizers*. Basic Books; 2008.
13 Woods G. Mother's Little Helpers. *British Journal of Psychiatry*. 2018; 208(6): 555.
14 Keefe P. *Empire of Pain*. Knopf Doubleday; 1921.
15 Intelligence P. https://pink.citeline.com/PS008594/PURDUE-FREDRICK-WILL-SUBMIT-NDA-FOR-MS-CONTIN.
16 Meier B. Opioid's Maker Hid Knowledge Of Wide Abuse. *New York Times*. May 29, 2018. www.nytimes.com/2018/05/29/health/purdue-opioids-oxycontin.html.
17 Non-Dependence USf. The Role of Opioids in Treating Postsurgical Pain. 2022. www.planagainstpain.com/resources/usnd/.
18 Greenfield SF, Back SE, Lawson K, Brady KT. Substance Abuse in Women. *Psychiatric Clinics of North America*. June 2010; 33(2): 339–355. doi:10.1016/j.psc.2010.01.004.
19 Kelly JP, Cook SF, Kaufman DW, Anderson T, Rosenberg L, Mitchell AA. Prevalence and Characteristics of Opioid Use in the US Adult Population. *Pain*. September 15, 2008; 138(3): 507–513. doi:10.1016/j.pain.2008.01.027.
20 Campbell CI, Weisner C, Leresche L, et al. Age and Gender Trends in Long-term Opioid Analgesic Use for Noncancer Pain. *American Journal of Public Health*. December 2010; 100(12): 2541–2547. doi:10.2105/ajph.2009.180646.
21 Pharmacological Management of Persistent Pain in Older Persons. *Pain Medicine*. September 2009; 10(6): 1062–1083. doi:10.1111/j.1526-4637.2009.00699.x.
22 Robeznieks A. Women Bear Greater Burden of Opioid Epidemic. American Medical Association. June 27, 2018. www.ama-assn.org/delivering-care/overdose-epidemic/women-bear-greater-burden-opioid-epidemic.
23 Unruh AM. Gender Variations in Clinical Pain Experience. *Pain*. May to June 1996; 65(2–3): 123–167. doi:10.1016/0304-3959(95)00214-6.

24 Greenfield SF, Brooks AJ, Gordon SM, et al. Substance Abuse Treatment Entry, Retention, and Outcome in Women: A Review of the Literature. *Drug and Alcohol Dependence.* January 5, 2007; 86(1): 1–21. doi:10.1016/j.drugalcdep.2006.05.012.

25 Bougie, O, Blom, J, Zhou, G, Jurji, A, Thurston, J. Use and Misuse of Opioid After Gynecologic Surgery. *Best Practice & Research Clinical Obstetrics and Gynaecology.* 2022; 85(22): 23–24.

26 Statistics NCfH. Births-method of Delivery 2021. Centers for Disease Control. www. cdc.gov/nchs/fastats/delivery.htm.

27 Bateman BT, Franklin JM, Bykov K, et al. Persistent Opioid Use Following Cesarean Delivery: Patterns and Predictors Among Opioid-naïve Women. *American Journal of Obstetrics and Gynecology.* September 2016; 215(3): 353.e1–353.e18. doi:10.1016/j.ajog.2016.03.016.

28 Health OoWs. Hysterectomy. U.S. Government. December 29, 2022. www.women-shealth.gov/a-z-topics/hysterectomy.

29 Lie AK, Hansen H, Herzberg D, et al. The Harms of Constructing Addiction as a Chronic, Relapsing Brain Disease. *American Journal of Public Health.* April 2022; 112(S2): S104–s108. doi:10.2105/ajph.2021.306645.

30 Stein MD, Anderson BJ, Kenney SR, Bailey GL. Beliefs About the Consequences of Using Benzodiazepines Among Persons with Opioid Use Disorder. *Journal of Substance Abuse Treatment.* June 2017; 77: 67–71. doi:10.1016/j.jsat.2017.03.002.

31 Paulozzi LJ, Strickler GK, Kreiner PW, Koris CM. Controlled Substance Prescribing Patterns—Prescription Behavior Surveillance System, Eight States, 2013. *MMWR Surveillance Summary.* October 16. 2015; 64(9): 1–14. doi:10.15585/mmwr. ss6409a1.

32 Torres-Bondia F, Dakterzada F, Galván L, et al. Benzodiazepine and Z-Drug Use and the Risk of Developing Dementia. *International Journal of Neuropsychopharmacology.* April 19, 2022; 25(4): 261–268. doi:10.1093/ijnp/pyab073.

33 Fine DR, Herzberg D, Wakeman SE. Societal Biases, Institutional Discrimination, and Trends in Opioid Use in the USA. *Journal of General Internal Medicine.* March 2021; 36(3): 797–801. doi:10.1007/s11606-020-05974-0.

34 Drug Policy Alliance. Framework: Building Black Feminist Visions to End the Drug War. 2023. https://drugpolicy.org/wp-content/uploads/2023/12/black-feminist-visions-NoBleed.pdf.

35 Report TC. *A Tragic Link: Drugs and Rising Women's Incarceration.* The Crime Report. https://thecrimereport.org/2020/11/10/a-tragic-link-drugs-and-rising-womens-incarceration/.

36 Ryan HG, Glover, S. OxyContin Goes Global—"We're Only Just Getting Started." *Los Angeles Times.* December 18, 2016. www.latimes.com/projects/la-me-oxycontin-part3/.

4

UNDER THE INFLUENCE

Pharmaceutical Relationships and Their Impact on Endometriosis Care

Heather Guidone

> Federal law protects patients from medical providers who write prescriptions
> so they can enrich themselves, and from drug companies who do not play by
> the rules in their marketing and promotional efforts.
> (United States Attorney William M. McSwain, October 26, 2018)[1]

Clinically defined as the presence of endometrial-like tissue in extra-uterine sites,[2] endometriosis is a heterogeneous, systemic inflammatory disease affecting an estimated 190 million women and girls and unmeasured amounts of transgender and gender-expansive individuals globally.[3,4,5,6] The disease results in distorted pelvic anatomy, adhesions, inflammation, endometriomas, fibrosis, and other problems[7] leading to pain and symptoms that may become chronic. Treatments range from symptom-directed (i.e., medical suppression), to removal of the disease itself via surgery. There is no definitive cure, and pathogenesis remains the subject of spirited debate.

Endometriosis is a major cause of pain, subfertility, disability, and significantly compromised quality of life and is commonly associated with impaired bowel, urinary, sexual, and reproductive functions (i.e., dysmenorrhea, cyclic and acyclic pain, dysuria, dyschezia, dyspareunia, and infertility, and much more).[8] Although commonly gynecologic in nature, extra-pelvic disease has been reported in a "considerable number" of cases[9] and, indeed, the full effects of endometriosis go "far beyond the pelvis."[10]

The disease is also frequently associated with various and significant comorbidities that may contribute to the fact that endometriosis remains fundamentally mired in outdated assumptions. Much of what is communicated about the

DOI: 10.4324/9781003472711-5

disease reflects a stagnant belief system that confounds the diagnostic and treatment processes and leads to poor health outcomes for many.

Despite its prevalence, the disease remains subject to lengthy diagnostic delays up to a decade or even longer following symptom onset. Even once a diagnosis is established, a distinct lack of standardized clinical guidelines results in inconsistent management, with medical menstrual suppression, hysterectomy, and pregnancy still too frequently recommended as "definitive" care.

These failing standards leave those struggling under-resourced and exposed to conflicting information about best practices, and the landscape of care is vulnerable to potential industry influence. Much of the guidance towards "treatments" is authored by contributors with financial ties to the pharmaceutical industry, with potential benefits of timely surgery often missing from this guidance.

To be certain, people need equitable access to life-changing, life-saving drug therapies and devices. Research must continue to develop valuable new drugs and products and make them accessible to all those who would benefit. At the same time, there is a growing demand for transparency and unbiased, patient-centered care based on truly evidence-based guidelines. This chapter explores the potentially harmful impacts of partnerships between pharmaceutical companies and advocacy groups, physicians, scientists, and others in the endometriosis space. While such collaborations may have advantageous results, it is also true that these alliances do not always benefit the patients they purport to represent and serve.

Endometriosis Then and Now

A substantive review of the history of endometriosis is outside the scope of this chapter; however, early references to endometriosis-type symptoms have been described at least as far back as 1500 BC in the Ebers Papyrus.[11] Nezhat and colleagues[12] further detailed the presence of probable endometriosis in early medical writings dated over 4,000 years ago in their extraordinary and exhaustive review, "Endometriosis: Ancient Disease, Ancient Treatments." The authors suggest there is further irrefutable evidence that "hysteria, the now discredited mystery disorder presumed for centuries to be psychological in origin, was most likely endometriosis in the majority of cases," and as Jones[13] further proposes, discourse about endometriosis is "at least related to if not influenced by the social forces that shaped a diagnosis of hysteria."

While Carl Freiherr von Rokitansky is credited with first describing the scientific and histological aspects of the disease in 1860,[14,15] it is Albany, NY gynecologist John Sampson, MD who is recognized for "naming" endometriosis and upon whose 1927 theory of retrograde menstruation[16] much of the disease discourse is still based, despite having been challenged and even clarified over the past century.

The disease is among the leading causes of gynecologic hospitalization in just the United States (US) alone,[17] and it imposes a direct and indirect cost burden of nearly $70 million annually on the American healthcare system as of 2018.[18] Data from all major countries has demonstrated that endometriosis is a more costly public health problem than much more publicly acknowledged conditions (e.g., migraine and Crohn's), and its prevalence is similar to that of type II diabetes and rheumatoid arthritis.[19,20]

Unfortunately, much of what is communicated about the disease reflects an outmoded belief system that complicates the diagnostic and treatment processes and can lead to poor outcomes. Myths and misinformation are spread widely, with some of the most prominent and vocal organizations promoting inaccuracies; consequently, the media routinely describe endometriosis incorrectly. As a direct result, the disease is erroneously minimized as merely a "menstrual condition" or "normal" period pain resulting from "endometrium gone rogue." In fact, the ectopic "lesions" of endometriosis resemble but are not identical to the normal endometrium.[21] It has been well documented how the lesions differ functionally from their native counterpart and feature an abundance of differential invasive, adhesive, and proliferative behaviors.[22,23,24,25,26] Research continues to improve understanding of the genetics and genomics of the disease, furthering knowledge of endometriosis biology.[27]

Endometriosis has been found in every major organ system, including far-distant extra-pelvic locations like the lungs, spleen, and even, rarely, the brain.[28,29] Diagnosis is considered definitive when endometriosis lesions are confirmed via surgical biopsy.[30,31,32] Histopathological analysis requires the presence of at least two of the following: epithelium, glands, stroma, and/or hemosiderin-filled macrophages.[33] Although it is a priority research focus, no clinically relevant, non-invasive biomarkers are available outside the bench setting as yet; similarly, no medication response "confirms" a diagnosis. A combination of history, physical examination, and/or laboratory/diagnostic/imaging studies can help eliminate non-endometriosis concerns and are important for presurgical planning, yet such approaches are highly operator-dependent and often have poor sensitivity, specificity, and predictive value. Most importantly, these findings cannot constitute diagnostic confirmation in many cases.

Although classically viewed (in error) by many as merely a "disease of menstruation," possessing a uterus and experiencing menses are not requisite to diagnosis. Endometriosis has been documented in post-hysterectomy,[34,35] post-menopausal,[36,37,38,39,40] and other non-menstruating individuals, rarely in those assigned male at birth,[41] among trans- and gender-nonconforming individuals,[42,43,44,45,46] and in the human fetus.[47,48,49] Yet despite all evidence to the contrary, many sources continue to frame the disease as simply "painful periods" easily treated through menstrual suppression, despite its profound, body-wide impact.

Subsequent to the antiquated notion of endometriosis as merely "killer cramps," menstrual suppression, hysterectomy, and even pregnancy are frequently recommended as "definitive" care, despite having little influence on the disease itself. Endometriosis has major systemic implications and is frequently diagnosed concomitantly with various better-recognized comorbidities.[50,51,52] Such diagnoses include but are not limited to gastrointestinal and/or bladder dysfunction, gynepathologies like adenomyosis and fibroids, certain autoimmune diseases, allergies, asthma, fibromyalgia, chronic fatigue, rheumatoid arthritis, coronary heart disease, slightly increased risks of certain cancers, and stroke.

Unfortunately, although modern medical knowledge, clinical experience, and therapies are ever-evolving, endometriosis remains fundamentally mired in outdated and false assumptions. Treatment guidelines, often based on conflicting information, leave those struggling with the disease under-resourced and vulnerable to conflicting information about best practices. Moreover, the field of endometriosis care remains exposed and vulnerable to the potential pitfalls of industry influence.

As noted above, people need equitable access to life-changing—in many cases life-saving—drug therapies and medical products. Specifically, medical therapy may be the preferred or even sole option for many living with endometriosis, and it should remain widely accessible. Researchers absolutely must continue to develop clinically valuable new drugs and devices and make them affordable. At the same time, transparent and unbiased treatment guidelines must also be a priority.

The average new drug costs between $500 million and 1+ billion and takes up to two decades to develop. Corporations have an obvious and even understandable self-interest in reducing the likelihood of failure and increasing potential revenue. Simply, they must consider whether the amount of money spent to get a drug to market will be less than the drug's anticipated revenue across the patent exclusivity lifetime.[53] Potential returns are lucrative; the endometriosis drug market is currently valued at nearly $711 million, with global growth projected towards a staggering $2.9 billion by 2027. The economic forecast is, as expected, centered on pharmaceutical options (i.e., gonadotropin-releasing hormone (GnRH) analogs and other suppressive therapies).[54]

In their 2018 landmark paper, Fabbri and colleagues[55] wrote: "Industry-sponsored studies tend to be biased in favor of the sponsor's products. Several studies have explored this issue, documenting how the funding source can influence the design, conduct, and publication of research." While the authors performed their comprehensive review to identify and synthesize studies exploring the influence of industry sponsorship on research agendas across different fields, not singularly on endometriosis, their findings are applicable to endometriosis drug research.

Endometriosis Organizations and Pharma: Integral Community Partners with Conflicts of Interest?

Broadly speaking, partnerships between patient and professional organizations and industry partners are not problematic per se. Such collaborations may help shape research directions, increase funding, and lead to developments that improve lives. When the collaboration influences the disease narrative, dictates care in a way that benefits the sponsor and enriches the charity but does not improve the lives of patients, or leads to limitations rather than expansion in care access, however, such alliances constitute conflicts of interest.

Pharmaceutical corporations will often work with community-based programs on a "philanthropic" basis to increase access to care and provide other beneficial services to healthcare consumers. Patient advocacy groups frequently collaborate with industry to increase incentives for investment in disease-specific programs. There is growing concern, however, that industry support for these groups is not as altruistic as it would appear. Corporate and community partnerships are often aimed more towards the benefit of the company.

The potential influence of so-called "big pharma" on advocacy groups is a growing area of investigation. At least one study found that organizations receiving pharma support in turn often vocally endorsed or echoed the manufacturer's position, while groups that had received minimal financing instead focused their advocacy on the drug's side effects.[56] Other more recent reports indicate that some patient groups with ties to industry essentially "endorse" the company's talking points, allow the company access to their member lists for the purposes of direct marketing, permit data mining of the charity's patient information, and even enlist their patient members (on pharma's dime) in support of various product campaigns.[57] Another recent Swedish study[58] found that while patient organizations frequently collaborate with drug companies, such partnership can result in concerns about commercial agendas influencing patient advocacy.

Other authors investigating the lack of transparency by patient advocacy groups that fail to fully disclose the amount of drug company funding they receive even called some of these groups "tools of the pharmaceutical industry,"[59,60] noting that "many appear unable or unwilling to take positions on consumer issues such as lowering prescription drug prices that might anger their drug corporation funders."

Others have sounded the alarm over the recent trend of joint coalitions being formed between patient groups and pharma, usually completely funded by the industry partner. Such groups can potentially "amplify the company's messaging and even allow for drugmakers to influence policy without proper disclosures."[61] As Susannah Rose, PhD, Scientific Director of Research, Office of

Patient Experience at the Cleveland Clinic, stated: "Those communities are also stocked with potential policy advocates. And with no disclosure requirements, it's often impossible to know whether drugmakers' contributions are shaping the patient groups' policy stances."

Perhaps this troubling lack of transparency and potential influence is most eloquently summed up by Dr Matthew McCoy,[62] lead author of a paper published in *The New England Journal of Medicine* critiquing the murky financial relationships between patient/advocacy organizations and drug, device, and related industry corporations: "The 'patient' voice is speaking with a pharma accent"—as is the likely intention.

Among the most prominent of industry influencers in the endometriosis space include Myovant, acquired in 2023 for the hefty sum of $2.9 billion to become a wholly owned subsidiary of Sumitomo Pharma,[63] and AbbVie, Inc., the research-based pharmaceutical spinoff of Abbott, Inc. Neither company is a stranger to financial support of various charities, including those established specifically to benefit patients with endometriosis.

In August 2022, the US Food & Drug Administration (FDA) granted approval for Pfizer and Myovant Sciences' relugolix 40mg, estradiol 1mg, and norethindrone acetate 0.5mg drug, Myfembree®, to "manage moderate to severe pain linked with endometriosis in pre-menopausal women."[64] The company prides itself on "transformative advocacy" by funding "vital projects and partnering with passionate leaders to redefine care in women's health," including endometriosis. [65] One might question, then, whether this "redefining of care" is a push towards widespread use of its GnRH antagonist, relugolix (the company's answer to AbbVie's Orilissa®). The company has a history of supporting various health initiatives and events, including those for or related to the disease (e.g., Voices of Periods,[66] Female Forward Together,[67] HealthyWomen,[68] the Society of Endometriosis & Uterine Disorders,[69] the Women's Health Innovation Summit,[70] AAGL,[71] and many others). More recently, the company also sponsored the Endometriosis Foundation of America's 2023 "Patient Day" symposium,[72] and has a permanent page on the organization's website at https://www.endofound.org/-/myovant.[66]

To its credit, Myovant is known for sponsoring heretofore underfunded initiatives in the Inclusion, Diversity, and Equity space; less transparent, however, is how much support is actually provided to the various platforms, unlike competitor AbbVie which provides full public accounting. Myovant undoubtedly engages in such initiatives in an endeavor to provide equitable, charitable support to worthy causes. The company's hard push to ensure the inclusion of Myfembree® in practice guidelines, including those of the American College of Gynecology (ACOG), American Society for Reproductive Medicine (ASRM), American Association of Gynecologic Laparoscopists (AAGL), or other country-specific guidelines,[73] however, is ostensibly a deciding factor as to which organizations the company chooses to support. Endorsement (real or perceived) of their product by influential societal bodies within endometriosis and reproductive health communities is critical to their success, as their product(s) "need to be included or positioned favorably in such treatment guidelines and pathways" lest the "full utilization potential of [their] products may not be reached, which may harm [the company's] ability to successfully commercialize [their] current or any future approved products."[73] Additionally, supporting inclusive patient organizations is one way companies can demonstrate corporate social responsibility to investors.

For its part, AbbVie donated $24.7 million to 59 patient groups in just 2015 alone.[74] From its founding in 2013 through year-end 2021, the company donated over $30 million to various organizations either related directly to endometriosis care or those concerned with medical education at least peripherally related to the disease. To date, over $550,000 of the $30 million went to just five endometriosis charities in the forms of "charitable donations, corporate sponsorships, educational grants, and patient support."[75–86]

Endometriosis Association	$160,000.00
Endometriosis Foundation of America	$42,500.00
Fundacion Puertorriquena DE Pacientes Consult Endometriosis	$37,960.00
World Endometriosis Research Foundation	$18,000.00
World Endometriosis Society	$300,000.00

One might wonder whether such generous support for these organizations, particularly prior to 2019, was done out of charitable spirit and not in anticipation of garnering support and public endorsement for the company's then-forthcoming endometriosis drug.

AbbVie officially became a company on January 1, 2013 in separation from Abbott, the healthcare conglomerate which was formerly part of the joint venture TAP created by Takeda and Abbott Pharmaceuticals in 1977. TAP was one of the most successful joint ventures in the history of American business; in 2007, the company had revenues of $3.1 billion from just two marketed products alone, Prevacid® and Lupron®, the latter of which has been long promoted as a treatment for endometriosis-associated symptoms.[87]

Incidentally, TAP later pleaded guilty to criminal conspiracy for providing physicians with free samples of Lupron® throughout the 1990s, for which Medicare was billed. The resulting settlement in 2001 represented the largest to that date, with the company paying out $290 million in criminal fines, $559 million to the federal government, and $25.5 million to the states. Combined with TAP's related $150 million Racketeer Influenced & Corrupt Organizations Act (RICO) settlement with patients and private insurers in 2004, the overall payout to settle the various lawsuits relating to the company's sales tactics (which included charges of conspiracy to pay "kickbacks," often classified as "educational grants," to physicians if they prescribed Lupron®) was over $1 billion.[88,89] This was not the last of the company's legal entanglements related to drug promotion. In May 2012, Abbott pleaded guilty and agreed to pay $1.5 billion to settle accusations about its promotion of Depakote® for uses not approved by the FDA.[90] Abbott Laboratories and AbbVie also paid $25 million in 2018 to "resolve allegations that it employed kickbacks and unlawful methods of marketing and promotion to induce physicians to prescribe the drug TriCor®."[91]

In mid-May 2021, AbbVie became the subject of a hearing by the US House of Representatives Committee on Oversight and Reform, which reviewed the company's pricing and business practices.[92] At the hearing centered on the ongoing drug-pricing crisis, Congresswoman Katie Porter leveled scathing criticism against AbbVie's Chairman of the Board and Chief Executive Officer, Richard Gonzalez, stating: "You're feeding us lies that we must pay astronomical prices to get innovative treatments." Porter contrasted AbbVie's litigation and settlements expenses from 2013 to 2018 ($1.6 billion) and $4 billion annual marketing and advertising expenses with the "mere" $2.45 billion spent on research and development.[93] Incidentally, Mr. Gonzalez' own salary package in 2021 was $23.9 million.[94]

In 2010 (pre-AbbVie spinoff), Abbott also entered into a highly profitable collaboration with Neurocrine Biosciences to develop and commercialize the GnRH antagonist elagolix for the treatment of endometriosis-related pain (with intention for use in treating fibroids as well). With an upfront payment to Neurocrine of $75 million and Abbott's funding of all development activities, the collaboration was expected to net additional milestones and payouts exceeding $575 million. Abbott was to hold worldwide exclusive rights to the drug under the agreement. With Lupron® coming off patent in 2015, elagolix represented a blockbuster for Abbott and subsequently the AbbVie spinoff. AbbVie, founded soon afterwards, primarily addressed six areas: hepatitis C, neuroscience, immunology, oncology, renal disease, and women's health. AbbVie needed the new product to remain a leader in the endometriosis market.

On July 24, 2018, the United States (US) Food & Drug Administration approved elagolix, branded as Orilissa®. Administered as a daily pill, the GnRH antagonist is indicated for "the management of moderate to severe pain associated with endometriosis."[95] AbbVie states[95,96] that Orilissa® can cause serious side effects, including bone mineral density loss that may not be completely reversible; altered menstrual bleeding that may reduce the ability to recognize pregnancy; hepatic transaminase elevations; hot flushes and night sweats; headache; nausea; insomnia; amenorrhea; anxiety; arthralgia, new onset or worsening depression, anxiety, or other mood changes; depression-related adverse reactions and mood changes; and suicidal ideation and mood disorders. According to its literature, suicidal ideation and behavior, including one completed suicide, occurred in subjects treated with the drug in clinical trials. Likewise, patients in the trials taking the drug had a "higher incidence of depression and mood changes compared to placebo, and those with a history of suicidality or depression had a higher incidence of depression compared to patients without such history."[96] Orilissa® has also been associated with increased acute porphyric attacks in women with acute hepatic porphyrias (AHPs) and should be avoided, or used with caution, in patients with AHPs.[97]

In 2018, an analysis conducted by The Institute for Clinical and Economic Review (ICER), an independent non-profit research institute that produces evidence reports on the effectiveness and value of drugs, also determined that "elagolix show[ed] promise in reducing the pain women with endometriosis experience (particularly in those with dysmenorrhea or menstrual-related pain), but more research is needed to determine the drug's long-term effectiveness and safety profile, particularly in comparison to alternative agents" and that "there is insufficient evidence to rule out the possibility of treatment-related harms."[98]

Yet vigorous promotion of Orilissa® accompanied the drug's roll-out, including prime-time television ads and infinite numbers of on- and off-line materials. One physician publicly announced that the drug could even "avert surgical complications" and encouraged its use vs. operative intervention, tagging his "viral" post "#surgeryinapill," much to the dismay of the endometriosis community of patients and practitioners alike, who responded swiftly to clarify the error of such a claim.[99] AbbVie did not respond with any clarification. Incidentally, that physician "Tweet" author received over 1,031 industry payments overall from 2015 to 2021, totaling $557,937.88. Some 394 payments totaling $251,394.85 were from AbbVie specifically in the form of non-research compensation. The bulk of the AbbVie payments was received by this physician in 2019—the year of the company's ramped-up marketing efforts for Orilissa®.[100]

Generally, endometriosis organizations and industry-affiliated physicians and researchers exercise at least some caution in publicly endorsing any particular therapies for the disease. However, in one widely circulated interview on EndometriosisNews.com at the time regarding the drug, the Founder of the Endometriosis Foundation of America (EFA) called the FDA's approval of Orilissa® "truly incredible news," lending support (real or perceived) to AbbVie's assertion that Orilissa® "represents a significant advancement for women with endometriosis and physicians who need more options for the medical management of this disease."[101] His organization received a $30,000 corporate sponsorship from AbbVie that year.

Eight months later in response to vocal feedback at their 2019 annual meeting, it was subsequently announced that "two $10,000 checks from AbbVie had in fact been returned."[102] However, AbbVie donated $42,500 overall to EFA, with pre-spinoff Abbott having made at least one additional prior sponsorship donation in 2010 of approximately $10,000.[103,104] To the best of this author's knowledge and belief, no mention of return of that total amount has been made.

To be certain, endometriosis non-profit support overall is infinitesimal compared to other disease organizations' receipts (e.g., the Crohn's & Colitis Foundation Inc. has received more than $2.7 million from AbbVie). Endometriosis remains under-supported on all fronts, even charitable donations. Nevertheless, in addition to the company's still-generous fiscal support of various endometriosis non-profits, the "Alliance for Endometriosis" was founded at the company's expense in 2020.

The "Alliance for Endometriosis" is a collaborative venture between AbbVie and ACOG, the Endometriosis Association, Black Women's Health Imperative, GE Healthcare, HealthyWomen, and the International Pelvic Pain Society. One Alliance spokesperson, who has also served as an AbbVie consultant, described the mission as an effort to "expand the conversation, build awareness and education, reduce stigma and facilitate communication ... so that the women who are impacted by this disease can receive proper and efficient care."[105]

Sponsored by AbbVie and developed in consultation with Alliance members, the initiative features a patient-facing survey and resources such as a link to "finding a doctor," which redirects to AbbVie's SpeakEndo™ website.[106] That secondary's site's privacy policy, which redirects again to AbbVie corporate, indicates that it collects personal data used by the company to "provide marketing communications that promote the use of or offer participation in AbbVie products, services, programs, research events or provide other information that may be of interest." The policy further states, "In some cases, we collect your Personal Data with your consent. In other cases, we collect this information for our legitimate business interest to optimize and customize AbbVie Relationships." The company also details how it shares that personal data "with third parties, such as name, address, date of birth, gender, address, phone number, financial information related to qualification in certain income-based and financial support programs, including your social security number or national identification number (where permitted or required by law), sensitive data such as health data relating to your disease or condition, medical history, treatment, reason for discontinuation, data on active management of the disease and insurance coverage and benefits related to your use of our products."[107] At its launch, the SpeakEndo™ site encouraged patients to sign up to the platform despite the fairly invasive information collection process by broadly advertising that "for every person who signs up, a donation will be made to the Endometriosis Foundation of America" (and later "to the Endometriosis Association"). From 2013 through 2021, Alliance member IPPS received $163,000 in "charitable donations, corporate sponsorships, and educational grants" from AbbVie. The Endometriosis Association received $160,000 in charitable donations from the company.

The Alliance's materials are problematic in that they incorrectly describe endometriosis as "a disease where the tissue that forms the inside lining of the uterus grows where it doesn't belong—sometimes on the ovaries, fallopian tubes and other organs found in the pelvic area," reinforcing the erroneous belief that native endometrium and endometriosis are identical and that the disease is primarily reproductive in nature. "Common symptoms" are listed as "swelling and period pain, as well as pain throughout the month and during sex," with no mention of the systemic impact of the disease.[108] ACOG, once described by famed gynecologic surgeon Harry Reich, MD as having "expressed little interest in surgery for this disease" along with doubtful interest in "ever wanting to help patients with endometriosis" but a solid interest in "wanting to help big pharma" and from which "all endometriosis surgeons should resign in mass (sic),"[109] received $436,350 from AbbVie in the form of "corporate sponsorships and educational grants."

The organization's own endometriosis guidelines largely and unsurprisingly eschew surgical intervention, promoting both initial drug therapy and empiric retreatment with additional suppressive medications, citing the rationale of "inherent risks and imprecision of surgery for definitive diagnosis" as well as suppression post-surgically.[110] No mention of any "inherent risks" of any drugs used for endometriosis or widespread complaints from the global patient community about side effects are included. Moreover, the ACOG Guidelines, which were reaffirmed in 2018 but have not been updated since 2010, have themselves been the subject of ardent advocacy efforts. Unfortunately, when implored by advocates to support substantive updates to the Guidelines, the then-Vice President of Health Policy at ACOG called such efforts "naïve."

It is unclear what if any financial support Black Women's Health Imperative has received from AbbVie, though the organization lists the company among its "partners" at https://bwhi.org/partners. HealthyWomen, which features "AbbVie supported" content,[111] hosts AbbVie on its Corporate Advisory Council, and lists the company among its funders.[112] The organization's CEO is also prominently featured among AbbVie's "stories."[113]

Alliance member GE Healthcare is a company specializing (in part) in medical imaging and which sponsors the DEFEND (Developing an Ultrasound-MRI-biomarker fusion model for Endometriosis) study. The company promotes imaging "diagnosis" for endometriosis and features such sentiments on its website[114,115] as "we should be moving away from surgery." Without surgical intervention, one assumes then that the company's recommended approach to the disease must be to "treat" endometriosis through medical suppression (i.e., Orilissa® or other drugs).

The Society for Women's Health Research (SWHR), which received $275,015 from AbbVie through 2021, has also partnered with the company. The Society produced "an Endometriosis Toolkit" through its "Endometriosis & Fibroids

Network" with the company's support. The Toolkit encourages "taking hormonal therapy after surgery...[to] eliminate or delay the return" of the disease and asserts that "experts" are moving away from surgical intervention towards "less invasive treatment options, such as the medication, hormonal therapies," [116] further promoting the drug therapy narrative and discouraging access to surgical intervention for those who may benefit from it. No mention is made of the fact that drug therapy is intended only (and is FDA approved) for temporary relief of pain associated with endometriosis, not actual treatment of the disease. Nor is there mention of the expense or vast side effect profiles that often result in lack of adherence and discontinuation of therapy.

The SWHR organization has also hosted a related AbbVie-sponsored endometriosis roundtable featuring several prominent researchers and physicians, many of whom also serve/have served as AbbVie consultants.[117] That event led to an academic publication in *The American Journal of Obstetrics and Gynecology (AJOG)* on unmet needs in endometriosis.[118] While that expert review does indicate that surgical intervention remains the gold standard, it upholds the recommendation of "many experts in the field" that "definitive diagnosis is not always required before initiating medical therapy," thereby amplifying the position of limiting "diagnosis" and "treatment" of endometriosis to non-surgical interventions. Supported by a programmatic grant from AbbVie, 40% of the authors were/are consultants to, and/or serve on the International Advisory Board of, and/or receive(d) research funding from, and/or were/are a member of the speaker's bureau for AbbVie. Similarly, 25% of The SWHR Interdisciplinary Network on Endometriosis and Fibroids contributors were/are consultants to, and/or serve on the International Advisory Board of, and/or receive(d) research funding from the company.[116] To its credit, as of this writing, the Society has continued its work to expand more neutral/inclusive endometriosis education and policy improvements by hosting diverse Working Group efforts and "Day on the Hill" activities.

The World Endometriosis Society and the World Endometriosis Research Foundation have also received support in the amount of at least a combined $318,000 from AbbVie. Each organization features multiple "board members" and/or "ambassadors" with strong industry ties. Author disclosures such as "received honoraria for advice to" AbbVie; "served as consultant" for AbbVie; "received personal fees from" (AbbVie, Bayer, Merck, Myovant, Bayer, and Merck); "received grants from" AstraZeneca and Ferring; "received consulting fees from" Nordic Pharma illustrate and underscore the heavy financial ties between the pharmaceutical industry and individuals representing these organizations. Note that such disclosures do not appear on the organizations' websites.[119,120] Indeed, such financial relationships in isolation are not necessarily problematic; however, many of the same individuals have collaborated with other industry-funded authors, including the writing of various treatment guidelines.

Among the most recent guidelines include those by the European Society of Human Reproduction and Embryology (ESHRE), current revisions to which now recommend withholding surgery for diagnosis and treatment altogether, except "in patients with negative imaging results and/or where empirical treatment was unsuccessful or inappropriate."[121] Essentially, medical suppression, administered even without a definitive diagnosis, is largely "required" before a patient might be subsequently referred to surgery—no matter how severe their disease may potentially be. Many of the contributors have financial ties to pharma and device companies; one highly influential author remains a vocal critic of surgery for endometriosis. This is not unexpected, given that he has a patent pending on a serum endometriosis biomarker promoted as useful for "non-invasive diagnosis and has multiple pharmaceutical relationships.[122]

Bayer Pharma subsequently unveiled their own Guidelines for diagnosis and early management of endometriosis in Asia in 2022, with strong recommendation for "clinical diagnosis and early medical therapy." Unsurprisingly, the company states their Guidelines "were in alignment with those published by [ESHRE]."[123]

The Australian guidelines feature those authored in part by collaborators who also served or currently serve as pharma consultants to Bayer, Merck, and various other industry members.[124] As with similar materials, the recommendations lean heavily towards pharmaceutical intervention and do not characterize any differences between excision vs. ablation when discussing surgery for the disease, citing "lack of evidence" despite conflicting findings by other authors.

Upon publication, the Australian guidelines were broadcast around the global media with headlines widely proclaiming "You No Longer Need Surgery to be Diagnosed with Endometriosis."[125] Negative reaction from the patient community to these guidelines was so widespread across countless social media campaigns that it prompted a formal response from the committee Chair.[126] The Chair later went on to characterize opposing views to the guidelines under the "Ugly" category of his editorial during Endometriosis Awareness Month, which is paywalled in a journal of which he is Deputy Editor, calling patient and advocacy response concerning the hormonal treatment of endometriosis and differing surgical techniques "vitriolic"—which he later quietly changed to "passionate."[127] The Chair is also on the advisory board of Gedeon Richter Plc., a European multinational pharmaceutical and biotechnology company headquartered in Budapest.

Australia is no stranger to controversy in endometriosis. Previously, then-Health Minister Greg Hunt publicly apologized in 2017 on behalf of the Australian government for the delay in diagnosis and lack of treatment for endometriosis, which was a declaration without precedent. Hunt also introduced a national action plan and additional funding. More recently, Hunt and Prime Minister Scott Morrison announced a record $58 million to be provided under the plan for access to "funded MRIs, research scholarships, a digital platform to access evidence-based disease information, and educational programs." It is not clear what funds if any will be used to implement increased physician training on the disease or to fund access to gold-standard endometriosis care for patients.[128]

Despite the ongoing persuasive push solely towards drug suppression, at least one recent study on the treatment of endometriosis from New Zealand found that "hormonal medications were often considered ineffective, but were routinely offered as the first, or only, options for patients."[129] Some patients in that study reported that delaying surgery caused long-lasting damage, including threat to their fertility.[130] One American celebrity even sued her insurer over lack of care for her disease, citing ineffective treatment with birth control pills and her medically documented need for surgical treatment.[131] She was denied coverage because her health plan determined that such treatment was "infertility related" and therefore not covered. The parties later reached a settlement, and her settlement was based on her physical and emotional suffering.

Several studies have documented how the funding source can influence the design, conduct, and publication of research. Although more difficult to define, sponsorship can also influence the research agenda.[55] As Breault and Knafl noted in their 2020 review, "physician participation in company-funded trials is essential to medical progress."[132] Physician-researchers can become experts on the drugs being studied and are often invited to join the sponsor's speaker's bureaus, advisory committees, boards of directors, and other collaboratives, and they may receive compensation for doing so. Such financial interactions "can be viewed as potential conflicts of interest."[132]

While there are laws and ethics guidelines in place to regulate conflicts of interest in medical research, some scientists have noted that:

> Investigators with conflicts of interest are more likely to arrive at positive conclusions, perhaps as a result of biased study design, industry suppression of negative results, preferential funding by industry of projects that are likely to succeed, or biased interpretation of results on the part of investigators.[133]

Ensuring the integrity of research (and preserving trust in the profession) are critical. When the participation of leading physicians and/or academicians in certain research endeavors leads to real or perceived support of a product or device, their influence may limit options for care—and it is patients who suffer. The development and marketing of elagolix provides a relevant example of partnerships between industry and academia.

Seventeen of the 25 most cited articles on endometriosis treatment (the majority written on elagolix) were authored largely by AbbVie employees. Of those authors not directly employed by the company, one Yale researcher[134] is notable for strong financial ties to AbbVie. He has authored no less than 15 pro-Orilissa® studies openly arguing for use of "empiric medical therapy prior to laparoscopy in the diagnostic and treatment algorithm unless fertility is a priority" (presumably valuing procreative potential over quality of life). He received $95,541.35 via 108 general payments from AbbVie along with $6,259.54 and $186,512.82 in associated research funding, for a total of $288,313.71 from 2015 to 2021.[100] Another leading endometriosis researcher serves on AbbVie's International Advisory Board and has secured millions in research grants/funding from the company.[135] In addition, she is also affiliated with an academic hospital that received $1,412,690 from AbbVie from 2013 to 2021 in the form of Fellowships and/or Educational Grants.[75–86]

Elagolix, Research, and Endometriosis

As noted earlier in this chapter, industry funds industry research, and biomedical companies routinely partner with academic/research support to investigate, develop, and bring their product to market. Industry-sponsored research "tends to be biased in favor of the sponsor's products,"[55] and while there is generally nothing nefarious about such R&D collaborations at face value, such partnerships potentially deprive patients of access to multiple treatment considerations.

Pharma has been accused of "furthering its own ends by various means such as expedient trial design and presentation of data, suppression of unfavorable findings, regulatory capture, ghostwriting, funding of continuing medical education and marketing of off-label drug use."[136] As authors Angell and Seymour-Relman[137] wrote: "Many clinical trials are never published because the results do not favor the sponsor's product. There have been several widely publicized cases of investigators who published negative results anyway and were harassed by their industry sponsors for doing so."

The field of gynecology research is not immune to such influence or pressure. Other researchers have lamented the general lack of pharma's openness in research and clinical trials on endometriosis, calling for increased transparency regarding selective publication and the suppression of unfavorable (to industry) findings from clinical trials funded by drug companies.[138]

Media Messages: The Face of Endometriosis—or the Face of Pharma?

It is not just organizations or healthcare professionals who lend support to pro-pharma messaging on treatments. As part of its Orilissa®-oriented promotional campaign, AbbVie recruited actor, singer, and *Dancing with the Stars* champion Julianne Hough to "SpeakEndo™" as their paid spokesperson. A deep dive into the campaign by famed journalist Jessica Meiselman found that the ties were not so transparent, however, writing that the company "did not disclose Hough's material connection to AbbVie" and, in those articles which did offer mention of the relationship, the campaign did so without clarity of origin, instead noting that Hough was the "face of … a national campaign aimed at spreading aware-ness of the condition." The author further found that other articles positioned Hough as merely "a spokesperson for SpeakEndo™, an organization that raises awareness about endometriosis and endometriosis symptoms, which could be construed as a kind of community outreach or charity work"[139] rather than a paid agent of AbbVie.

Hough's is not the first celebrity face to endorse drug therapy for endometrio-sis. The Hough campaign is reminiscent of Abbott's early Lupron® promotions featuring model, MTV VJ, actor, and *New York Times* bestselling author Karen "Duff" Duffy. In her role as "official spokesperson for the disease," Duffy, who was "controlling her endometriosis with Lupron®" at the time, reported "no side effects from the drug,"[140] an experience that represented a stark contrast to the side effects reported by many Lupron® users.

In a subsequent trend, "Patient Influencers" have also become targets for various industry partnerships. The term "Patient Influencer" is defined as "those who promote pharmaceutical medications and/or medical devices, allowing companies to leverage the patient experience and expertise in the design, devel-opment and promotion of their products and services."[141]

While there are "legal requirements in place surrounding direct to consumer communications, including FDA regulations to ensure communications are ac-curate and backed by evidence, social media influence continues to have gray areas."[142] By "building relationships directly with patients using covert persua-sion tactics like partnering with social media influencers," some companies have launched an effort to improve the negative perceptions of pharma across the healthcare consumer landscape. Indeed, studies have shown that "digital opin-ion leaders" are well positioned and able to "change the attitudes of their fol-lowers, increase acceptance of the information provided, and even influence the intention to buy corresponding products."[143]

Further described by authors Butler and Fugh-Berman[144] as "patients who have gained trust and stature within a patient community," such individuals "speak as everyday people with medical conditions, as relatable as a friend from high school." Partnerships with industry may include such services as "pro-ducing videos and other content, attending events, providing advice, and even recruiting patients for industry-funded clinical studies"—all without having to disclose sponsor ties. The authors note the danger of non-disclosure when bol-stering and broadcasting the views of a corporate entity with its own incentives and allegiances:

> Patient leaders, who have built their trusted communities without any outside resources, revenue from—and warm relationships with—industry may in fact influence what they believe, because the relationship reinforces industry-friendly opinions, creates the illusion of partnership, and lessens the chances that patients will adopt industry-critical stances.

Physicians and Pharma

From 2016–2021, AbbVie paid $448,855,519 (4,329,392 payments) in general payments and $1,499,180,632 (204,735 payments) in research payments to physicians, non-physician practitioners, and teaching hospitals for a total of $1,948,036,151. Nearly half the payments were for consulting services. Dr. Robert Alpern, the previous Dean of Yale School of Medicine, is among the top recipients of both AbbVie and Abbott, having received 199 payments between 2016–2021 totaling $3,474,116.[100]

Endometriosis-dedicated physicians, including gynecologic surgeons, are also heavily involved with industry, including pharma (which may seem surprising given that the latter's primary income is presumably surgical in nature). For example, one highly regarded endometriosis and "Minimally Invasive Gynecologic Surgeon" (MIG) is high on the AbbVie recipient list, having received 1,207 payments in compensation totaling $858,650. Another MIG surgeon, an extremely popular social media personality with millions of content views, received $55,533 via 123 payments. Another self-proclaimed "gyn influencer" received $448,306 via 582 general payments and 4 research payments totaling $13,750. Another prominent surgeon and head of a prestigious New York City academic MIGS program received $41,393 via 61 general payments and 4 research payments totaling $12,952. Another of the country's leading robotic endometriosis and MIG surgeons, received $244,525 (388 payments). This small sampling gives an indication that even those purporting to lean towards surgical intervention for the disease have complex relationships with AbbVie, one of the most influential pharmaceutical companies in the endometriosis space.[100]

Professional organizations often rely heavily on industry benefactors as well; to be certain, this is not problematic in and of itself. However, such sponsorship may have a *quid pro quo* effect. For example, as outlined on AbbVie's public accounting of the company's grants and donations, the pharmaceutical giant paid $276,550 in corporate sponsorships to the leading international organization "dedicated to Elevating Gynecologic Surgery" between 2017 and 2021. That organization in turn featured prominent advertising and facilitated numerous AbbVie-sponsored sessions throughout its international meetings. Among others on the hefty disclosure list, AbbVie also provided $133,800 in corporate sponsorship to the "leading organization for the science and practice of reproductive medicine" from 2017 to 2021. The company was again in turn prominently featured throughout various physician-facing meetings. Perhaps more concerning, however, is the sponsorship of physician education resources. For example, WebMD and Medscape (part of the WebMD Health Professional Network), leading sources of physician education, have received $13,455,799 and $13,120,784 respectively between 2013 and 2021; both websites feature extensive AbbVie-supported materials.[145,146]

There are recommendations in place for industry sponsorship of medical societies and their educational events to be kept to a minimum and openly declared on societies' websites and in materials, yet heavy sponsorship plays out in meetings and online every day. These activities invariably translate into patient care that is influenced by pharma.[136]

Legislating Industry Support—Congress and Pharma

Although outside the scope of this chapter, legislators are also recipients of sizable donations from industry. For example, although they "do not provide political contributions in anticipation of, in recognition of, or in return for an official act,"[147] from 2007 to 2022, AbbVie made $3,778,250 in campaign contributions.[148] Specifically, contributions from the AbbVie PAC in 2021/2022 to federal candidates (51.07% to Democrats, 48.49% to Republicans) totaled $562,000.[149] While some contributions were in the realm of what constitutes a pittance ($12; Tammy Baldwin, Candidate D-WIS1), others such as those to Mitch McConnell (R-KYS1, one of the top pharma recipients overall) were more substantial ($12,413). McConnell, who has been accused of sabotaging bipartisan drug-pricing bills that would benefit the American people,[150] is followed by close second Brad Schneider (Candidate D-IL10) at $11,000 for the cycle.

Campaign contributions to members of Congress overall are familiar territory for pharma. From 2013 to 2021, AbbVie contributed $3,778,250 to legislators, with only a single Representative (John Rose, R-TN) reporting zero dollars in contributions. Top recipients include the following:[148]

Rep. Kevin McCarthy (R CA)	$75,000
Sen. Mitch McConnell (R KY)	$57,500
Rep. Steve Scalise (R LA)	$56,000
Rep. Patrick McHenry (R NC)	$47,500
Rep. Steny Hoyer (D MD)	$44,500
Rep. Anna Eshoo (D CA)	$44,000
Sen. Christopher Coons (D DE)	$43,500
Sen. Patty Murray (D WA)	$42,500
Rep. Scott Peters (D CA)	$41,500

Pharma-sponsored activities can affect how doctors practice medicine.[151] From the non-profit setting to research to physicians to policy work to editorial boards to political campaigns, pharma influence across the endometriosis landscape is pervasive. Many of those who are receiving fiscal compensation from pharma and/or have lent perceived support to a particular product or device often in turn create guidelines and policies influencing treatment guidelines.

These guidelines are considered standards of care, yet it is undeniable that they increasingly convey a "less laparoscopy, more hormone therapy"[152] sentiment with the consequence of more patients losing access to *multidisciplinary treatment choices.*

Conclusions

Endometriosis is a systemic, multifaceted disease requiring multidimensional approaches to care. Yet as Vercellini and colleagues[153] noted,

> a stepped-care approach is certainly not in the interest of the eight pharma industries that are currently developing GnRH antagonists for endometriosis because resorting to these medications only in cases of failure of first-line treatments would imply a drastic reduction of revenues.

Nevertheless, management of the disease must incorporate *all*—combined, even—options and consider at its center the patient's preferences, priorities, and desired outcomes. Yet this is not the overarching message conveyed by the various guidelines that ostensibly represent evidence-based standards of care.

To make educated, empowered decisions, patients must be informed of all potential benefits, harms, costs, and expected outcomes of all management options. This is the sacred construct of informed consent. Endometriosis management options must not be limited to those preferred by the provider, whether the reason is the provider's limited surgical skill or bias resulting from the influence of pharma. To wit, "The physician should be able to look the patient in the eye and explain in detail all the available treatments—not only those that the physician prefers or is able to offer."[154] Patients do not often know how industry relationships may be shaping professional views on endometriosis care or whether there are other options not offered by a particular provider. The same holds true for patient-facing organizations who are often relied upon to provide accurate, unbiased endometriosis education, yet may instead be promoting sponsor-driven materials.

This is certainly not to suggest that ethical breaches are the norm in legislative–industry–gynecology–charity partnerships. It is undeniable, however, that the standard of care for those suffering from endometriosis publicly promoted and favored by many thought leaders on the disease, some of whom hold highly lucrative financial ties to industry, is pharmaceutical intervention. At the same time, pharma lobbies legislators to protect drug pricing and policies that benefit the industry, and this, too, limits options for optimal, integrative care.

There are no easy answers for endometriosis. Absent definitive cure(s) and better treatments, the disease needs more management options, including medical, and, better, affordable access to all care choices, including surgery.

The primary objective of any collaborations between industry and academia, medicine, legislators, and the non-profit sector must largely be to benefit patients—not to benefit of the recipients of grants, fundings, donations, honoraria, or other support.

Access to quality care for endometriosis is already fraught by disparities, and the growing promotion of drug suppression as the sole diagnostic and therapeutic intervention is not in the best interest of patients. Hindering access to *any* option and offering only suppression vs. surgery or vice versa—a practice not based on robust evidence or patient-centered priorities—is unacceptable. As Mijatovic and Vercellini wrote,[155] the result is vulnerable patients who are "more likely to accept the suggestions of their healthcare provider, which can lead to unbalanced and physician-centered decisions ... in favor of either medical or surgical treatment"—when in fact long-term disease management is far more comprehensive and multidisciplinary. Judicious, timely referrals to appropriate subspecialists who can offer best practices must not be obstructed by those who are controlling the disease narrative towards a single-minded agenda.

PRIMUM NON NOCERE.[156]

Notes

1 United States Attorney William M. McSwain for the United States Department of Justice, U.S. Attorney's Office, Eastern District of Pennsylvania. October 26, 2018. "Abbott Laboratories and AbbVie Inc. to Pay $25 Million to Resolve False Claims Act Allegations of Kickbacks and Off-Label Marketing of the Drug TriCor®." Web: www.justice.gov/usao-edpa/pr/abbott-laboratories-and-AbbVie-inc-pay-25-million-resolve-false-claims-act-allegations. Accessed November 1, 2021.

2 International Working Group of AAGL, ESGE, ESHRE and WES, Tomassetti C, Johnson NP, Petrozza J, Abrao MS, Einarsson JI, Horne AW, Lee TTM, Missmer S, Vermeulen N, Zondervan KT, Grimbizis G, De Wilde RL. An International Terminology for Endometriosis, 2021. *Journal of Minimally Invasive Gynecology*. November 2021; 28(11): 18491859.

3 Zondervan KT, Becker CM, Missmer SA. Endometriosis. *New England Journal of Medicine*. March 26, 2020; 382(13): 1244–1256.

4 Saunders PTK, Horne AW. Endometriosis: Etiology, Pathobiology, and Therapeutic Prospects. *Cell*. May 27, 2021; 184(11): 2807–2824.

5 Brunty S, Mitchell B, Bou-Zgheib N, Santanam N. Endometriosis and Ovarian Cancer Risk, an Epigenetic Connection. *Annals of Translational Medicine*. December 2020; 8(24): 1715.

6 Jones CE. Queering Gendered Disabilities. *Journal of Lesbian Studies*. 2021; 25(3): 195–211.

7 Yong PJ, Bedaiwy MA, Alotaibi F, Anglesio MS. Pathogenesis of Bowel Endometriosis. *Best Practice and Research. Clinical Obstetrics and Gynaecology*. March 2021; 71: 2–13.

8 Gruber TM, Mechsner S. Pathogenesis of Endometriosis: The Origin of Pain and Subfertility. *Cells*. June 3, 2021; 10(6): 1381.

9 Andres MP, Arcoverde FVL, Souza CCC, Fernandes LFC, Abrão MS, Kho RM. Extrapelvic Endometriosis: A Systematic Review. *Journal of Minimally Invasive Gynecology*. February 2020; 27(2): 373–389.

10 Taylor HS, Kotlyar AM, Flores VA. Endometriosis Is a Chronic Systemic Disease: Clinical Challenges and Novel Innovations. *The Lancet.* February 27, 2021; 397(10276): 839–852.

11 Acién P, Velasco I. Endometriosis: A Disease that Remains Enigmatic. *ISRN Obstetrics and Gynecology.* July 17, 2013: 242149.

12 Nezhat C, Nezhat F, Nezhat C. Endometriosis: Ancient Disease, Ancient Treatments. *Fertility and Sterility.* December 2012; 98(6 Suppl): S1–62.

13 Jones CE. Wandering Wombs and "Female Troubles": The Hysterical Origins, Symptoms, and Treatments of Endometriosis. 2015. *Women's Studies;* 44(8): 1083–1113.

14 Batt RE. *A History of Endometriosis.* London, Springer Verlag, 2011. ISBN 978-0-85729-585-9.

15 Batt RE. Invited comment on the paper by Benagiano et al., The History of Endometriosis. *Gynecologic and Obstetric Investigation.* 2014; 78(1): 10–11.

16 Chaichian S. It Is the Time to Treat Endometriosis Based on Pathophysiology. *Journal of Reproductive Infertility.* January–March 2019; 20(1): 1–2.

17 McLeod BS, Retzloff MG. Epidemiology of Endometriosis: An Assessment of Risk Factors. Clinical Obstetrics and Gynecology. June 2010; 53(2): 389–396.

18 Soliman AM, Surrey E, Bonafede M, Nelson JK, Castelli-Haley J. Real-world Evaluation of Direct and Indirect Economic Burden among Endometriosis Patients in the United States. *Advances in Therapy.* 2018; 35(3): 408–423.

19 Fourquet J, Gao X, Zavala D, Orengo JC, Abac S, Ruiz A, Laboy J, Flores I. Patients' Report on How Endometriosis Affects Health, Work, and Daily Life. *Fertility and Sterility.* May 1, 2010; 93(7): 2424–2428.

20 Zondervan K, Becker CM, Missmer S. Endometriosis. *New England Journal of Medicine.* 2020; 382: 1244–1256.

21 Ahn SH, Khalaj K, Young SL, Lessey BA, Koti M, Tayade C. Immune-inflammation Gene Signatures in Endometriosis Patients. *Fertility and Sterility.* November 2016; 106(6):1420–1431.e7.de.

22 Zanatta A, Rocha AM, Carvalho F, Pereira R, Taylor HS, Motta E, Baracat E, Serafini P. The Role of the Hoxa10/HOXA10 Gene in the Etiology of Endometriosis and its Related Infertility: A Review. *Journal of Assisted Reproduction and Genetics.* 2010; 27(12): 701–710.

23 Freger S, Leonardi M, Foster WG. Exosomes and Their Cargo Are Important Regulators of Cell Function in Endometriosis. *Reproductive Biomedicine Online.* June 3, 2021: S1472-6483(21)00281-9.

24 Fonseca MAS, Haro M, Wright KN, Lin X, Abbasi F, Sun J, Hernandez L, Orr NL, Hong J, Choi-Kuaea Y, Maluf HM, Balzer BL, Fishburn A, Hickey R, Cass I, Goodridge HS, Truong M, Wang Y, Pisarska MD, Dinh HQ, El-Naggar A, Huntsman DG, Anglesio MS, Goodman MT, Medeiros F, Siedhoff M, Lawrenson K. Single-cell Transcriptomic Analysis of Endometriosis. *Nature Genetics.* January 9, 2023.

25 Jiao L, Wang J, Zhu L. A Comparative Study of Endometriosis and Normal Endometrium Based on Ultrasound Observation. *Applied Bionics and Biomechanics.* April 30, 2022: 793469.

26 Delbandi AA, Mahmoudi M, Shervin A, Akbari E, Jeddi-Tehrani M, Sankian M, Kazemnejad S, Zarnani AH. Eutopic and Ectopic Stromal Cells from Patients with Endometriosis Exhibit Differential Invasive, Adhesive, and Proliferative Behavior. *Fertility and Sterility.* September 2013; 100(3): 761–769.

27 Hansen KA, Eyster KM. Genetics and Genomics of Endometriosis. *Clinical Obstetrics and Gynecology.* June 2010;53(2): 403–412.

28 Weyl A, Illac C, Delchier M-C, Suc B, Cuellar E, Chantalat E. Splenic Lesion Mimicking Breast Metastasis: The First Description of Splenic Parenchymal Endometriosis. *Journal of Endometriosis and Pelvic Pain Disorders.* 2021; 13(1): 69–73.

29 Asally R, Markham R, Manconi F. Endometriosis–Pathogenesis and Sequelae. *Journal of Reproductive Medicine and Gynecological Obstetrics*. 2018, 3: 010.

30 Saunders PTK, Horne AW. Endometriosis: Etiology, Pathobiology, and Therapeutic Prospects. *Cell*. May 27, 2021; 184(11): 2807–2824.

31 Laudański P, Rogalska G, Warzecha D, Lipa M, Mańka G, Kiecka M, Spaczyński R, Piekarski P, Banaszewska B, Jakimiuk A, Issat T, Rokita W, Młodawski J, Szubert M, Sieroszewski P, Raba G, Szczupak K, Kluz T, Kluza M, Neuman T, Adler P, Peterson H, Salumets A, Wielgos M. Autoantibody Screening of Plasma and Peritoneal Fluid of Patients with Endometriosis. *Human Reproduction*. February 7, 2023: dead011.

32 Signorile PG, Cassano M, Viceconte R, Spyrou M, Marcattilj V, Baldi A. Endometriosis: A Retrospective Analysis on Diagnostic Data in a Cohort of 4,401 Patients. *In Vivo*. January/February 2022; 36(1): 430–438.

33 Wang T, Jiang R, Yao Y, Qian L, Zhao Y, Huang X. Identification of Endometriosis-associated Genes and Pathways Based on Bioinformatic Analysis. *Medicine (Baltimore)*. July 9, 2021; 100(27): e26530.

34 Rizk B, Fischer AS, Lotfy HA, Turki R, Zahed HA, Malik R et al. Recurrence of Endometriosis After Hysterectomy. *Facts, Views and Vision in Obgyn*. 2014; 6(4): 219–227.

35 Mathey MP, Bouquet de Jolinière J, Major A, Pugin F, Monnard E, Fiche M, Sandmeier D, Khomsi F, Feki A. Endometriotic Mass After Hysterectomy in a 61 Year Old Post-menopausal Woman: A Case Report and Update. *Frontiers in Surgery*. May 10, 2019;6: 14.

36 Secosan C, Balulescu L, Brasoveanu S, Balint O, Pirtea P, Dorin G, Pirtea L. Endometriosis in Menopause-renewed Attention on a Controversial Disease. *Diagnostics (Basel, Switzerland)*. February 29, 2020; 10(3):134.

37 Wasson MN. Chronic Pelvic Pain Caused by Postmenopausal Endometriosis. *Journal of Minimally Invasive Gynecology*. March/April 2020;27(3): 561–563.

38 Zhuang L, Eisinger D, Jaworski R. A Case of Ureteric Polypoid Endometriosis Presenting in a Post-menopausal Woman. *Pathology*. June 2017; 49(4): 441–444.

39 Ozyurek ES, Yoldemir T, Kalkan U. Surgical Challenges in the Treatment of Perimenopausal and Postmenopausal Endometriosis. *Climacteric*. August 2018; 21(4): 385–390.

40 Soliman AM, Du EX, Yang H, Wu EQ, Haley JC. Retreatment Rates Among Endometriosis Patients Undergoing Hysterectomy or Laparoscopy. *Journal of Women's Health (Larchmt)*. June 2017; 26(6): 644–654.

41 Makiyan Z. Endometriosis Origin from Primordial Germ Cells. *Organogenesis*. July 3, 2017; 13(3): 95–102.

42 Shim JY, Laufer MR, Grimstad FW. Dysmenorrhea and Endometriosis in Transgender Adolescents. *Journal of Pediatric and Adolescent Gynecology*. October 2020; 33(5): 524–528.

43 Rachlin K, Hansbury G, Seth T. Pardo S. Hysterectomy & Oophorectomy Experiences of Female-to-Male Transgender Individuals. *International Journal of Transgenderism*. 2010; 12: 3, 155–166.

44 Cook A, Hopton E. Endometriosis Presenting in a Transgender Male. *Journal of Minimally Invasive Gynecology*. 2017; 24: S126.

45 Ferrando CA, Chapman G, Pollard R. Preoperative Pain Symptoms and the Incidence of Endometriosis in Transgender Men Undergoing Hysterectomy for Gender Affirmation. *Journal of Minimally Invasive Gynecology*. January 2021; 23: S1553-4650(21)00051-0.

46 Ashley RT Yergens for the *Huffington Post*. Endometriosis and Gender Nonconformity. June 10, 2017. Web: www.huffpost.com/entry/pumpkin-spice-lattes-endo_b_10265178. Accessed November 1, 2021.

47 Schuster M, Mackeen DA. Fetal Endometriosis: A Case Report. *Fertility and Sterility*. January 2015; 103(1): 160–162.

48 Signorile PG, Baldi F, Bussani R, D'Armiento M, De Falco M, Boccellino M, Quagliuolo L, Baldi A. New Evidence of the Presence of Endometriosis in the Human Fetus. Reproductive Biomedicine Online. July 2010; 21(1): 142–147.

49 Signorile PG, Baldi F, Bussani R, Viceconte R, Bulzomi P, D'Armiento M, D'Avino A, Baldi A. Embryologic Origin of Endometriosis: Analysis of 101 Human Female Fetuses. *Journal of Cell Physiology*. April 2012; 227(4): 1653–1656.

50 Eoh KJ, Han M, Kim EH, Jung I, Kim YT. Markedly Increased Risk of Malignancies in Women with Endometriosis. *Gynecology and Oncology*. January 26, 2021: S0090–8258(21)00079–2.

51 Chen SF, Yang YC, Hsu CY, Shen YC. Risk of Rheumatoid Arthritis in Patients with Endometriosis: A Nationwide Population-based Cohort Study. *Journal of Women's Health*. 2021; 30(8): 1160–1164.

52 Farland LV, Degnan WJ 3rd, Bell ML, Kasner SE, Liberman AL, Shah DK, Rexrode KM, Missmer SA. Laparoscopically Confirmed Endometriosis and Risk of Incident Stroke: A Prospective Cohort Study. *Stroke*. October 2022; 53(10): 3116–3122.

53 Litterman NK, Rhee M, Swinney DC, Ekins S. Collaboration for Rare Disease Drug Discovery Research [Version 1; peer review: 2 approved]. F1000Research 2014; 3: 261 (https://doi.org/10.12688/f1000research.5564.1).

54 Global Newswire. Global Endometriosis Drugs Market to Reach $2.9 Billion by 2027. October 18, 2022. Web: https://tinyurl.com/4kdvvmw4. Accessed November 1, 2021.

55 Fabbri A, Lai A, Grundy Q, Bero LA. The Influence of Industry Sponsorship on the Research Agenda: A Scoping Review. *American Journal of Public Health*. November 2018; 108(11): e9–e16.

56 Pew Prescription Project. Persuading the Prescribers: Pharmaceutical Industry Marketing and its Influence on Physicians and Patients. November 11, 2013. Web:www.pewtrusts.org/en/research-and-analysis/fact-sheets/2013/11/11/persuading-the-prescribers-pharmaceutical-industry-marketing-and-its-influence-on-physicians-and-patients. Accessed November 1, 2021.

57 Kaiser Health News for NBC Universal. Patient Advocacy Groups Take in Millions from Drugmakers. Is There a Payback? April 8, 2018. Web: www.nbcnews.com/health/health-care/patient-advocacy-groups-take-millions-drugmakers-there-payback-n863486. Accessed November 1, 2021.

58 Mulinari S, Vilhelmsson A, Rickard E, Ozieranski P. Five Years of Pharmaceutical Industry Funding of Patient Organisations in Sweden: Cross-sectional Study of Companies, Patient Organisations and Drugs. *PLoS ONE*. 2020; 15(6): e0235021.

59 Reed T. Pharma's Influence on Patient Advocacy. *Axios*, June 30, 2021. Web: www.axios.com/2021/06/30/pharma-influence-patient-advocacy. Accessed November 1, 2021.

60 Patients for Affordable Drug. The Hidden Hand: Big Pharma's Influence on Patient Advocacy Groups. Web: https://patientsforaffordabledrugs.org/the-hidden-hand. Accessed November 1, 2021.

61 Ben Elgin for the *Los Angeles Times*. In its Fight to Keep Drug Prices High, Big Pharma Leans on Charities. April 29, 2019. Web: www.latimes.com/business/la-fi-drug-prices-charity-20190429-story.html. Accessed November 1, 2021.

62 McCoy MS, Carniol M, Chockley K, Urwin JW, Emanuel EJ, Schmidt H. Conflicts of Interest for Patient-advocacy Organizations. *New England Journal of Medicine*. March 2, 2017; 376(9): 880–885.

63 Alex Keown for BioSpace. Weeks after Rejecting First Offer, Myovant Agrees to Acquisition by Sumitovant. Web: www.biospace.com/article/weeks-after-rejecting-first-offer-myovant-agrees-to-acquisition-by-sumitovant. Accessed November 1, 2021.

64 Pharmaceutical Technology. US FDA Approves Pfizer-Myovant's Myfembree for Endometriosis Pain. August 8, 2022. Web: www.pharmaceutical-technology.com/news/fda-pfizer-myovant-myfembree. Accessed January 3, 2023.

65 Myovant www.myovant.com/our-advocacy/forward-together/#women.

66 Endometriosis Foundation of America. Web: www.endofound.org/-/myovant. Accessed March 29, 2023.

67 Myovant. Web: https://www.biospace.com/article/releases/female-forward-together-a-cross-sector-coalition-announced-to-advance-research-education-and-action-for-women-s-health/. Accessed March 29, 2023.

68 Myovant. Web: www.globenewswire.com/news-release/2021/02/16/2176189/0/en/HealthyWomen-and-Myovant-Sciences-Launch-Voices-of-Periods-to-Fight-Menstrual-Stigma.html. Accessed November 11, 2022.

69 SEUD. Web: https://seud.org. Accessed March 29, 2023.

70 Myovant. Web: https://event.on24.com/wcc/r/3544357/3142CA99D087BE57F2ED DBB1C9690A51. Accessed November 11, 2022.

71 AAGL. Web: https://foundation.aagl.org/donors. Accessed November 11, 2022.

72 Endometriosis Foundation of America. Web: www.endofound.org/opening-remarks-tracey-haas-do. Accessed March 29, 2023.

73 Myovant Sciences Ltd., Form 10-K filing, United States Securities and Exchange Commission, Washington, DC, 20549. In: Annual Report Pursuant to Section 13 or 15(d) of the Securities Exchange Act of 1934, for the fiscal year ended March 31, 2022. Commission file number 001-37929. Web: https://investors.myovant.com/static-files/19211dfb-20ac-47d2-ba73-73d07a580515. Accessed March 29, 2023.

74 Kaiser Health News. In: Prescription for Power Database. Web: https://khn.org/patient-advocacy/#company-8. Accessed November 11, 2022.

75 AbbVie Pharmaceuticals. Web: https://www.abbvie.com/content/dam/abbvie-dotcom/uploads/PDFs/2021-AbbVie-Grants-and-Contributions-Report.pdf.

76 AbbVie Pharmaceuticals. Web: https://www.AbbVie.com/content/dam/AbbVie-dotcom/uploads/PDFs/2020-AbbVie-Grants-and-Contributions-Report.pdf.

77 AbbVie Pharmaceuticals. AbbVie has apparently taken down reports for the earlier years. The original links are recorded accurately. Web: www.AbbVie.com/content/dam/AbbVie-dotcom/uploads/PDFs/2019-AbbVie-Grants-and-Contributions-Report.pdf.

78 AbbVie Pharmaceuticals. AbbVie has apparently taken down reports for the earlier years. The original links are recorded accurately. Web: www.AbbVie.com/content/dam/AbbVie-dotcom/uploads/PDFs/2018-AbbVie-Grants-and-Contributions-Report.pdf.

79 AbbVie Pharmaceuticals. AbbVie has apparently taken down reports for the earlier years. The original links are recorded accurately. Web: www.AbbVie.com/content/dam/AbbVie-dotcom/uploads/PDFs/2017-AbbVie-Grants-and-Contributions-Report.pdf.

80 AbbVie Pharmaceuticals. AbbVie has apparently taken down reports for the earlier years. The original links are recorded accurately. Web: www.AbbVie.com/content/dam/AbbVie-dotcom/uploads/PDFs/2015-AbbVie-Grants-and-Contributions.pdf.

81 AbbVie Pharmaceuticals. AbbVie has apparently taken down reports for the earlier years. The original links are recorded accurately. Web: www.AbbVie.com/content/dam/AbbVie-dotcom/uploads/PDFs/2015-AbbVie-Grants-and-Contributions.pdf.

82 AbbVie Pharmaceuticals. AbbVie has apparently taken down reports for the earlier years. The original links are recorded accurately. Web: www.AbbVie.com/content/dam/AbbVie-dotcom/uploads/PDFs/2014-Grants-and-Contributions.pdf.

83 AbbVie Pharmaceuticals. AbbVie has apparently taken down reports for the earlier years. The original links are recorded accurately. Web: www.AbbVie.com/content/dam/AbbVie-dotcom/uploads/PDFs/1st_Quarter_2013_Grants_Donations_Report.pdf.

84 AbbVie Pharmaceuticals. AbbVie has apparently taken down reports for the earlier years. The original links are recorded accurately. Web: www.AbbVie.com/content/dam/AbbVie-dotcom/uploads/PDFs/FINAL_Q2-2013_Grants_and_Contributions_Posted_Document_07162014.pdf.

85 AbbVie Pharmaceuticals. AbbVie has apparently taken down reports for the earlier years. The original links are recorded accurately. Web: www.AbbVie.com/content/dam/AbbVie-dotcom/uploads/PDFs/AbbVie-2013-Q3-grants-donations.pdf.

86 AbbVie Pharmaceuticals. AbbVie has apparently taken down reports for the earlier years. The original links are recorded accurately. Web: www.AbbVie.com/content/dam/AbbVie-dotcom/uploads/PDFs/2013-Q4-2013-Grants-and-Contributions.pdf.

87 Takeda. Takeda, Abbott Announce Plans to Conclude TAP Joint Venture. March 18, 2008. Web: www.takeda.com/en-us/newsroom/news-releases/2008/takeda-abbott-announce-plans-to-conclude-tap-joint-venture/. Accessed November 11, 2022.

88 Melody Petersen for the *New York Times*. 2 Drug Makers to Pay $875 Million to Settle Fraud Case. October 4, 2001. Web: www.nytimes.com/2001/10/04/business/2-drug-makers-to-pay-875-million-to-settle-fraud-case.html. Accessed November 11, 2022.

89 Davis M. The Effects of False Claims Act Whistleblowers on the Pharmaceutical Industry. Harvard Law School, May 2006. Web: http://nrs.harvard.edu/urn-3:HUL. InstRepos:8965590. Accessed November 11, 2022.

90 Propublica data. Web: https://projects.propublica.org/d4d-archive/companies/AbbVie. Accessed November 11, 2022.

91 United States Attorney William M. McSwain for the United States Department of Justice, U.S. Attorney's Office, Eastern District of Pennsylvania. October 26, 2018. Abbott Laboratories and AbbVie Inc. to Pay $25 Million to Resolve False Claims Act Allegations of Kickbacks and Off-Label Marketing of the Drug TriCor®. Web: www.justice.gov/usao-edpa/pr/abbott-laboratories-and-AbbVie-inc-pay-25-million-resolve-false-claims-act-allegations. Accessed November 11, 2022.

92 Thomas Sullivan for Rockpointe Policy & Medicine, June 13, 2021. Web:www.policymed.com/2021/06/house-of-representatives-holds-hearing-focused-on-AbbVie-business-practices.html. Accessed November 11, 2022.

93 Tim Dickinson for *Rolling Stone Magazine*. Katie Porter Delivers Another Knockout Punch. May 19, 2021. Web: www.rollingstone.com/politics/politics-news/katie-porter-AbbVie-gonzalez-big-pharma-knockout-punch-1171735. Accessed November 11, 2022.

94 United States Securities & Exchange Commission, Washington, DC 20549. AbbVie, Proxy Statement Pursuant to Section 14(a) of the Securities Exchange Act of 1934. March 21, 2022, pp. 54. Web: https://investors.AbbVie.com/static-files/300d0981-6001-49f5-9f04-97960e5226e8. Accessed November 11, 2022.

95 AbbVie Pharmaceuticals. Web: www.rxAbbVie.com/pdf/orilissa_pi.pdf. Accessed November 11, 2022.

96 AbbVie Pharmaceuticals. Medication Guide, as approved by the U.S. Food and Drug Administration. Revised: February 2021. Web: www.rxAbbVie.com/pdf/orilissa_pi.pdf. Accessed November 11, 2022.

97 Ma CD, Bonkovsky HL. Elagolix is Porphyrogenic and May Induce Porphyric Attacks in Patients with the Acute Hepatic Porphyrias. *Molecular Genetics and Metabolism Reports*. September 7, 2022;33: 100915.

98 ICER. Institute for Clinical and Economic Review Report Questions the Adequacy of Evidence on Overall Health Benefit of Elagolix Given Limitations of Information on Safety and Limited Evidence Comparing to Other Treatment Options. June 15, 2018. Web: https://icer.org/news-insights/press-releases/endo-evidence-report. Accessed November 11, 2022.

99 Ian Taras, MD. December 9, 2019. Twitter: @DrTaras.

100 U.S. Centers for Medicare & Medicaid Services, Open Payments Database. Web: https://openpaymentsdata.cms.gov/company/100000000204. Web: https://open-paymentsdata.cms.gov/physician/66489

101 Larry Luxner for *Endometriosis News*. FDA Approves AbbVie's Orilissa to Treat Moderate to Severe Endometriosis Pain. July 24, 2018. Web: https://endometriosis-news.com/2018/07/24/fda-approves-AbbVies-orilissa-for-moderate-severe-endo-metriosis-pain. Accessed January 23, 2023.

102 Endometriosis Foundation of America. Web: www.endofound.org/dan-martin-david-redwine-great-debate-on-the-origins-of-endometriosis. Accessed November 11, 2022.

103 Endometriosis Foundation of America. Web: www.endofound.org/medical-confer-ence-2010-intro-1. Accessed November 11, 2022.

104 Personal correspondence between the author and the late Mark Burken, Abbott, 2010.

105 Bob Kronemyer for Contemporary Ob/Gyn. The Formation of the Alliance for Endometriosis. December 7, 2020. Web: www.contemporaryobgyn.net/view/the-formation-of-the-alliance-for-endometriosis. Accessed November 11, 2022.

106 AbbVie Pharmaceuticals. Web: www.speakendo.com/endometriosis-resources/doctor-locator. Accessed November 11, 2022.

107 AbbVie Pharmaceuticals. Web: https://privacy.AbbVie/privacy-policies/us-privacy-policy.html#information-parti-patient-cust-prog. Accessed November 11, 2022.

108 The Alliance for Endometriosis. The Alliance for Endometriosis Survey Reveals Actions Needed to Improve the Endometriosis Patient Experience. November 30, 2021. Web: www.prnewswire.com/news-releases/the-alliance-for-endometriosis-survey-reveals-actions-needed-to-improve-the-endometriosis-patient-experi-ence-301431226.html. Accessed November 11, 2022.

109 Harry Reich, MD, FACOG, FACS. Endometriosis: Hormonal or Surgical? My Reality! Breast, Ovary and Endometriosis: Endofound Medical Conference 2017. October 28, 2017. Lotte New York Palace Hotel. Web: www.endofound.org/endo-metriosis-hormonal-or-surgical-my-reality-harry-reich-md-facog-facs. Accessed November 11, 2022.

110 ACOG. Dysmenorrhea and Endometriosis in the Adolescent: ACOG Committee Opinion, Number 760, December 2018; American College of Obstetricians and Gynecologists (ACOG). Practice Bulletin #114: Management of Endometriosis. *Obstetrics and Gynecology*. July 2010; 116(1): 223–236, reaffirmed 2018.

111 HealthyWomen. Web: www.healthywomen.org/created-with-support/endometrio-sis. Accessed November 11, 2022.

112 HealthyWomen Annual Report, 2021. Web: https://roar-assets-auto.rbl.ms/docu-ments/17913/HW-2021-Annual-Report-FINAL.pdf?rand=1660245204237. Ac-cessed November 11, 2022.

113 AbbVie Pharmaceuticals. Web: https://stories.AbbVie.com/stories/evolving-endo-metriosis-conversation.htm. Accessed November 11, 2022.

114 GE Healthcare. Web: www.gehealthcare.com/insights/article/new-study-aims-to-revolutionize-the-diagnosis-of-endometriosis.

115 GE Healthcare. Web: www.gehealthcare.com/insights/article/one-in-ten-women-suffer-from-endometriosis-ultrasound-makes-diagnosis-faster-easier-and-safer. Ac-cessed March 13, 2023.

116 SWHR. 2021. Endometriosis Toolkit, A Patient Empowerment Guide. Web: https://swhr.org/wp-content/uploads/2021/03/SWHR_Endometriosis_Toolkit_3.2021.pdf. Accessed November 11, 2022.

117 SWHR Web: https://swhr.org/event/endometriosis-roundtable; https://swhr.org/event/endometriosis-shattering-misconceptions-shaping-the-future. Accessed No-vember 11, 2022.

118 As-Sanie S, Black R, Giudice LC, Gray Valbrun T, Gupta J, Jones B, Laufer MR, Milspaw AT, Missmer SA, Norman A, Taylor RN, Wallace K, Williams Z, Yong PJ, Nebel RA. Assessing Research Gaps and Unmet Needs in Endometriosis. *American Journal of Obstetrics and Gynecology*. August 2019; 221(2): 86–94.

119 World Endometriosis Research Foundation. Web: https://endometriosisfoundation. org/about/#board. Accessed November 11, 2022.

120 World Endometriosis Society. Web: https://endometriosis.ca/about. Accessed November 11, 2022.

121 Becker CM, Bokor A, Heikinheimo O, Horne A, Jansen F, Kiesel L, King K, Kvaskoff M, Nap A, Petersen K, Saridogan E, Tomassetti C, van Hanegem N, Vulliemoz N, Vermeulen N; ESHRE Endometriosis Guideline Group. ESHRE Guideline: Endometriosis. *Human Reproduction Open*. February 26, 2022; 2022(2): hoac009.

122 ESHRE. Funding/competing Interests. Web: https://academic.oup.com/hropen/article/2022/2/hoac009/6537540#authorNotesSectionTitle. Accessed November 11, 2022.

123 BioSpectrum Asia. March 4, 2022. Bayer Unveils Guideline for Diagnosis and Early Management for Endometriosis in Asia. Clinical Diagnosis and Early Medical Therapy. Web: https://www.biospectrumasia.com/news/30/19789/bayer-unveils-guideline-for-diagnosis-and-early-management-for-endometriosis-in-asia.html. Accessed November 11, 2022.

124 RANZCOG. 2021. Web: https://ranzcog.edu.au/news/australian-endometriosis-guideline. Accessed March 11, 2023.

125 Professor Mike Armour, Cecilia Ng, Dr Matthew Leonardi for The Conversation. You No Longer Need Surgery to Be Diagnosed with Endometriosis. June 6, 2022. Web: https://medicalxpress.com/news/2022-06-longer-surgery-endometriosis.html. Accessed November 11, 2022.

126 Professor Jason Abbott for the *Guardian*. Endometriosis Treatment in Australia Isn't Perfect–But There's a Lot to Celebrate. 29 March 2022. Web: www.theguardian.com/commentisfree/2022/mar/30/endometriosis-treatment-in-australia-isnt-perfect-but-theres-a-lot-to-celebrate. Accessed November 11, 2022.

127 Abbott JA. The Good, the Bad, and the Ugly of Endometriosis Guidelines. *Journal of Minimally Invasive Gynecology*. March 2023; 14: S1553–4650(23)00102-4.

128 Eda Tang for Stuff. Calls for Public Health Apology to Endometriosis Sufferers. March 26, 2022. Web: https://nzendo.org.nz/endo-news/calls-for-public-health-apology-to-endometriosis-sufferers%ef%bf%bc/. Accessed November 11, 2022.

129 Ellis K, Munro D, Wood R. The Experiences of Endometriosis Patients with Diagnosis and Treatment in New Zealand. *Frontiers in Global Womens Health*. August 31, 2022; 3: 991045.

130 Marie-Louise Connolly for the BBC. Endometriosis Surgery Delay "Caused Irreversible Damage." October 25, 2022. Web: www.bbc.com/news/uk-northern-ireland-63375713. Accessed November 11, 2022.

131 Jacklyn Wille for Bloomberg Law. Hilary Swank Settles Suit Over Health Coverage for Ovarian Cysts. August 9, 2021. Web: https://news.bloomberglaw.com/employee-benefits/hilary-swank-settles-suit-over-health-coverage-for-ovarian-cysts. Accessed November 11, 2022.

132 Breault J, Knafl E. Pitfalls and Safeguards in Industry-funded Research. *Ochsner Journal*. March 2020; 20(1): 104–110.

133 Okike K, Kocher MS, Mehlman CT, Bhandari M. Industry-sponsored Research. *Injury*. June 2008; 39(6): 666–680.

134 Agarwal SK, Chapron C, Giudice LC, Laufer MR, Leyland N, Missmer SA, Singh SS, Taylor HS. Clinical Diagnosis of Endometriosis: A Call to Action. *American Journal of Obstetrics and Gynecology*. April 2019; 220(4): 354.e1-354.e12.

135 Michigan State University. Unravelling the Causes and Consequences of Endometriosis: Stacey Missmer, ScD. *News Archives*. 2018. Web: https://obgyn.msu.edu/announcements/archive/2018/374-unravelling-the-causes-and-consequences-of-endometriosis-stacey-missmer-scd. Accessed November 11, 2022.
  Farquhar CM, Vercellini P, Marjoribanks J. Gynaecologists and Industry: Ain't No Sunshine. *Human Reproduction*. August 1, 2017; 32(8): 1543–1548.
136 AbbVie Pharmaceuticals. Web: https://www.abbvie.com/science/independent-educational-grants/grants-and-contribution-disclosures.html#:~:text=The%20list%20of%20AbbVie%E2%80%99s%20grants%20and%20contributions%20are,%24200%20from%20AbbVie%E2%80%99s%20US%20and%20Puerto%20Rico%20businesses.
137 Marcia Angell and Arnold Seymour-Relman for Daedalus. Patents, Profits & American Medicine: Conflicts of Interest in the Testing & Marketing of New Drugs. Spring 2022. Web: www.amacad.org/publication/patents-profits-american-medicine-conflicts-interest-testing-marketing-new-drugs. Accessed November 11, 2022.
138 Sun-Wei Guo for Endometriosis.org. Is There Transparency in Clinical Trials on Endometriosis? July 26, 2013. Web: https://endometriosis.org/news/opinion/is-there-transparency-in-clinical-trials-on-endometriosis. Accessed November 11, 2022.
139 Jessica Meiselman for *The Outline*. The Sneaky Way Pharmaceutical Companies Use Celebs to Market Their Drugs. April 15, 2019. Web: https://theoutline.com/post/7290/julianne-hough-abbvie-endometriosis-orilissa. Accessed November 11, 2022.
140 Susan Ferraro for *The New York Daily News*. Powering Through Pain. March 25, 2002. Web: https://www.nydailynews.com/2011/09/09/powering-through-pain/. Accessed November 11, 2022.
141 Willis E, Delbaere M. Patient Influencers: The Next Frontier in Direct-to-Consumer Pharmaceutical Marketing. *Journal of Medical Internet Research*. March 1, 2022; 24(3): e29422.
142 Dennis Thompson for *HealthDay News*. Patient Influencers on Social Media are Marketing Medicine, Devices. April 15, 2022. Web: www.upi.com/Health_News/2022/04/15/social-media-patient-influencers/9851650037117. Accessed November 11, 2022.
143 Metzler JM, Kalaitzopoulos DR, Burla L, Schaer G, Imesch P. Examining the Influence on Perceptions of Endometriosis via Analysis of Social Media Posts: Cross-sectional Study. *JMIR Formative Research*. 2022; 6(3): e31135.
144 Judy Butler and Adriane Fugh-Berman for *Health Affairs*. Patient Influencers Paid by Pharmaceutical Companies Should Be Required to Disclose Industry Ties. January 10, 2022. Web: www.healthaffairs.org/do/10.1377/forefront.20200109.985594/full. Accessed November 11, 2022.
145 Medscape. Web: www.medscape.org/viewarticle/964585. Accessed November 11, 2022.
146 WebMD. Web: www.webmd.com/women/endometriosis/news/20180724/fda-approves-new-drug-for-endometriosis-pain. Accessed November 11, 2022.
147 AbbVie Pharmaceuticals. Company Policies. Web: www.AbbVie.com/our-company/policies-disclosures.html. Accessed March 29, 2023.
148 Kaiser Health Network. Web: https://khn.org/news/campaign. Accessed November 11, 2022.
149 "The organizations themselves did not donate, rather the money came from the organizations' PACs, their individual members or employees or owners, and those individuals' immediate families. Organization totals include subsidiaries and affiliates."
  Open Secrets PAC Data. Web: www.opensecrets.org/political-action-committees-pacs/AbbVie-inc/C00536573/summary/2022. Accessed March 29, 2023.

150 Nicholas Florko for *Stat+ News*. Top Republican Blasts McConnell for Derailing Bipartisan Drug Pricing Bill. December 18, 2019. Web: www.statnews. com/2019/12/18/top-republican-blasts-mcconnell-for-derailing-bipartisan-drug-pricing-bill. Accessed March 29, 2023.
151 Lundh A, Lexchin J, Mintzes B, Schroll JB, Bero L. Industry Sponsorship and Research Outcome. *Cochrane Database of Systematic Reviews*. February 16, 2017; 2(2): MR000033.
152 Heidi Splete for Medscape. Updated Endometriosis Guidelines Emphasize Less Laparoscopy, More Hormone Therapy. February 8, 2022. Web: www.medscape. com/viewarticle/968117. Accessed November 11, 2022.
153 Vercellini P, Viganò P, Barbara G, Buggio L, Somigliana E. "Luigi Mangiagalli" Endometriosis Study Group. Elagolix for Endometriosis: All That Glitters Is Not Gold. *Human Reproduction*. February 1, 2019; 34(2): 193–199.
154 Vercellini P. Introduction: Management of Endometriosis: Moving Toward a Problem-oriented and Patient-centered Approach. *Fertility and Sterility*. 2015; 104(4): 761–763.
155 Mijatovic V, Vercellini P. Towards Comprehensive Management of Symptomatic Endometriosis: Beyond the Dichotomy of Medical Versus Surgical Treatment. *Human Reproduction*. January 10, 2024: dead262.
156 Latin, translated: "first, do no harm." In: "Of the Epidemics" as reviewed by Robert H. Shmerling, MD. First, Do No Harm. *Harvard Health Blog*. June 22, 2020. Web: www.health.harvard.edu/blog/first-do-no-harm-201510138421. Accessed November 11, 2022.

5

MENSTRUATION REPRESSION DISCOURSE IN ADVERTISEMENTS

An Ecofeminist Investigation

Anna Kubovski

Menstruation is a significant event in the lives of menstruators. It takes part in building their self-esteem and identity and influences their health, yet it remains a silenced topic in society. The use of the word "period" rather than "menstruation" emphasizes its perception as taboo. However, a prominent expression of menstruation in the public sphere is found in advertisements for menstrual products. Advertisements for menstrual products serve the feminine hygiene industry, estimated to be $47 billion in the global market in 2023, with annual growth of 5%.[1] One menstruator will use more than 11,000 disposable menstrual products (DMP)s in their lifetime.[2] The global feminine hygiene market has experienced significant growth and evolution in recent years, partly propelled by the popularity and profitability of disposable products. The market includes tampons, menstrual pads, menstrual cups, and vaginal health products.

The emphasis on effective advertising and marketing campaigns has played a pivotal role in the market's sustained growth. Advertisements have been instrumental in highlighting the convenience, absorbency, and discreetness of disposable feminine hygiene products. Numerous studies on menstrual discourse in advertisements reveal prominent discourses of shame and concealment, portraying menstruation as polluting and contemptible.[3,4] In parallel, another stream of advertising is scientific in nature, alongside representations of menstruators as physically active.[5,6] Among these studies, those that examine the representation of menstruation in Western society from an ecofeminist perspective are rare.

In this chapter, I use ecofeminist theory to explore common attitudes towards menstruation in Western society, which have constructed the inferiority of women compared to men and exposed the connection to the construction of

DOI: 10.4324/9781003472711-6

the female body and nature as inferior. I focus on the supposed inferiority of the female body and its representation in advertisements This kind of investigation allows a different observation on the representation of menstruation in advertisements, and the way they dictate what to think about the body and menstrual cycle. I demonstrate how capitalist consumer culture, together with the representation of menstruation in ads, preserves the alienation of women from their bodies, serves its construction as "other," and deviates from sociocultural norms, which causes harm to women's health.

Menstruation: General Background and the Construction of the "Other" Body

Traditional theories about menstruation have presented it as the reason for women's inferiority, mainly due to their physiological differences to men.[7,8,9] Due to her menstrual body, the woman was considered inferior to the man in her anatomy, psychology, and mental and intellectual abilities. The menstrual body is considered inferior to the female body when not menstruating and even more so to the male body. The connection between women and their bodies was strengthened through patriarchal perceptions and intensified with the help of science and the medical establishment.[10,11,12] The concept of women's inferiority due to their closeness to their body stems from the dichotomous thinking rooted in patriarchal Western thought, as revealed by ecofeminist theory.

Ecofeminist theory stands at the intersection of feminist and ecological thought. Ecofeminism posits that patriarchal hierarchies, which are implicated in the oppression of women, play a role in the domination of culture over nature. This domination leans on the philosophical dualism of differences, such as those between masculinity and femininity. In this duality, the masculine side is valued more highly than the feminine side.[13,14,15,16] The theory focuses on exposing the hierarchical division of "superior" and "inferior" groups and the social context in which superiors benefit from this unwarranted system.[17]

This dualist system creates, structures, and justifies the vitality and "naturalness" of control by superior groups over inferior groups. These dualisms reinforce characteristics of the superior side—such as men, culture, intellect, and the mind—being valued over the inferior side—such as women, nature, emotion, and the body. Moreover, female characteristics do not exist in their own right but only as opposites of their male counterparts. This system is used to justify women's political and intellectual subordination to men through the attribution of qualities such as passivity, weakness, and irrationality.[18] In this context, the body is perceived as a weakness, and because the woman is identified with the body, women are seen as negative, inferior, and uncontrollable.[14] The perception of this duality causes the woman to be seen as "other"; she exists only in comparison to the man. One key element in identifying the woman as other and connected to nature and the body is menstruation and the menstrual cycle.

Menstruation is a significant event in the lives of menstruators, contributing to building self-esteem, body image, and identity.[19] Through the years, the perception of menstruation has changed in Western societies. Menstruation has become a legitimate subject for discussion, under certain restrictions, including the sociocultural norms that define what is allowed to be said about menstruation and by whom, when, and where, known as "menstrual etiquette."[8] Yet there is still an almost entirely universal taboo surrounding menstruation, although different cultures and religions embed varied codes for coping with this taboo.[20] The menstruation taboo persists in its power today, even if perhaps only at a level of unconscious awareness.[21]

The perpetual taboo related to menstruation helps account for the burden of bodily shame that many menstruators experience. The emotion most associated with menstruation is shame, reinforced by social stigma.[22,23,24] This stigma contributes to the experience of negative feelings,[25] a tendency towards self-objectification,[18] self-body shaming,[26] and a negative body image,[27] which affects how menstruators perceive themselves and behave during menstruation.[28,29] Moreover, there is a negative social construction of menstruation as a nuisance. It is perceived as a dirty thing that causes pain and interferes with daily life.[28] These cultural norms, stigma, and taboos surrounding menstruation all create barriers to achieving menstrual health.[30,31]

Menstrual health is defined as the complete physical, mental, and social well-being of menstruators. Menstrual health is crucial for all menstruators' well-being, equality, rights, and dignity.[32] In terms of health and well-being, menstruation is incompletely understood medically.[33] Nowadays, there is a disregard in educational, sexual, and reproductive health programs, and menstruation is mostly addressed through a medical approach.[34] The menstrual cycle is treated as a health disorder that can be discussed in medical terms only and to which only medical solutions can be applied.[35] The medical discourse defines menstruation as a medical or even pathological event.[10] In addition, menstrual health problems tend to be normalized and dismissed, and menstruators often report delayed diagnoses and negative experiences when seeking institutionalized healthcare for menstrual-related issues.[36]

Under the auspices of medical discourse, the menstrual cycle and menstruation are controlled through medications to regulate and sometimes even stop menstruation. The use of the term "medication" promotes the perception that menstruation is a disease. This perception has popularized the current phenomenon of women controlling or suppressing their menstruation by using oral contraceptives such as the birth control pill.[37] Menstruation is treated as a disease and disability that requires constant supervision to keep from erupting. The accessibility of this type of control promotes menstrual concealment.[35]

"Feminine Hygiene" Products: Suppression of Menstruation Under the Auspices of Capitalism

The "feminine hygiene" industry serves as a powerful tool in the central discourse regarding menstruation and in constructing women as other in media and advertising. The female body is presented as other: mysterious, uncontrollable, threatening, seductive, and sexual. Due to this representation, the female body is seen as needing to be controlled—the industry relies on and benefits from that perception. The female body is shown in media and advertisements as inferior and defective and as finding comfort in the products.[38] Furthermore, the consumerist perspective links menstruation to illness or infection, and thus creates a link between femininity and infection, which engenders a view of menstrual blood as contaminating.[28]

Kimberly Clark was the first feminine care company to create advertisements for menstrual products with the sanitary napkins of Kotex in 1921.[39] Thousands of advertisements for menstrual products have since existed. Menstruation is conceptualized as a problem that can be solved by the consumption and use of DMPs, which are presented as the only solution for the menstruating body.[40,41] The medical industry, DMPs industry, and medical establishment are among the systems that profit from menstruation representation in advertisements.[28] Corporations are interested in maintaining the status quo because it ultimately sells their products in a fundamentally patriarchal society and marketplace.

In contemporary Western society, advertisements function as a significant agent in constructing reality. Advertisements play an important role in transmitting knowledge, messages, and meanings about menstruation, shaping and maintaining the prevalent perception. Advertisements for menstrual products convey the stigma surrounding it daily through various sociocultural structures. Menstruation is presented in advertisements as something to be hidden, ashamed of, and discouraged. Furthermore, using negative messages about menstruation is an effective way to market DMPs.[13] Advertisements for menstrual products use themes of secrecy and shame, and menstruation is frequently portrayed as a hygienic crisis that needs to be carefully managed through the advertised products.[42,43] At the same time, advertisements have been found to perpetuate common myths about and reinforce the taboo surrounding menstrual blood as a selling strategy.

Throughout the years, advertisements of menstrual products have tended to show highly objectified images of women or excluded images of women's bodies altogether.[41] This contributes to the sexualization of the female body, and women who internalize this cultural position often learn to feel disgust and shame towards the menstrual body.[27] The presentation of a single, sexualized body part, combined with the idealized depiction of the female form, reduces the woman to an object. The function of excluding women's bodies from advertisements is an attempt to provide a psychological buffer between the reproductive function of women's bodies and the cultural ideal of the objectified feminine body.[18]

The products marketed in the advertisements are disposable. The advertisements even highlight the convenience inherent in the one-time use of the product, which has become an indisputable norm. The consequences of the single-use trend are evident in the environment. They are embodied in an environmental cost that includes the depletion of natural resources, accumulation of waste, and nonperishable pollution.[44]

The capitalist consumer culture elevates single-use products, which are used and discarded carelessly without consideration for recycling. In addition, the normalization of single-use products allows the consumer to not consider the destructive impact consumption has on the environment.[45] In this way, the capitalist mechanism around menstruation is strengthened, which encourages the constant purchase of disposable products and suppression of the menstrual cycle.[46] It is evident that this culture, in which disposable products are used, works thanks to the dualism that connects femininity to nature and the body and treats these factors negatively or inferiorly to masculinity.

DMPs are also not beneficial to the body. Nowadays, there is no requirement for manufacturers of these products to disclose the materials their products are made from, although there are recommended[47,48,49] codes of practice for tampon manufacturers and distributors, which supposedly ensure a consistent approach to product labeling and consumer information on safety and correct use. Menstrual pads and tampons are made mainly from bleached cotton, nonwoven fabrics, and polymer absorbers; are not recyclable; and must be buried or incinerated. It takes 50 years for a pad to decompose; if burned, it is first chlorinated and disinfected.[50] Bleached pulp ingredients produce dioxins and other harmful substances that eventually enter the food cycle, polluting the environment and endangering natural species.[51] In addition, they may cause vulvovaginal candidiasis, itching, and even toxic shock syndrome.[52]

Analysis of Advertisements for Disposable Menstrual Products

Menstrual product advertising has preserved menstrual suppression and perpetuated the myths associated with menstruation and the menstrual cycle for decades. Given the fact that advertisements are among the most influential media globally,[53] and that they are one of the few arenas where public discourse around menstruation is acceptable, it is particularly important to examine their messages about menstruation. Analysis of advertisements allows for examining themes about menstruation, the female body, the status of women, and the perception of nature and how the use of these ideas increases sales of DMPs. Therefore, in the following sections, I examine the representation of menstruation and the female body in advertisements for menstrual products, exposing how the main themes are controlled by and, in turn, preserve Western society's mainstream approach.

One hundred unique menstrual product advertisements were collected (tampons, sanitary napkins, and pantyliners) of major companies in the field (Always, Kotex, Tampax, Carefree, Playtex, Bodyform, and O.B.) appearing on YouTube between October 2016 and January 2021. The advertisements were analyzed qualitatively using a phenomenologically oriented form of thematic analysis that draws from grounded theory while drawing from ecofeminist theory.[54,55] This technique offers the opportunity to obtain a comprehensive and clear understanding of the themes in the ads.

The collected advertisements were broadcast on television and uploaded to YouTube channels or broadcast directly between 1979 and 2021. The data were collected through a search engine using various keywords ("hygiene products," "menstrual products," "tampons," "sanitary napkin," "pantyliner," "pads," "feminine hygiene ads," "feminine hygiene products commercials," and "feminine hygiene products advertising") and company names (Always, Kotex, O.B., Tampax, Carefree, Alldays, Playtex, Bodyform, etc.). I have selected the ads of these companies because they are large Western manufacturers in the menstrual products market and transmit advertisements digitally.

I considered these advertisements as cultural texts representing the dominant ideology, exposing prevailing sociocultural norms. In the relevant context, advertisements are prominent in the public conversation surrounding menstruation, mainly because the taboo regarding this subject means that the messages conveyed through ads are usually the only public voice. It is crucial to analyze the messaging contained in these advertisements, because it represents the ruling discourse, helps construct it, and influences how menstruators experience their bodies and form their attitudes.

Several themes were found in ads throughout the selected time period, with multiple themes repeated at different times. Eight key themes emerged: (1) hiding, silencing, and shame; (2) safety and security; (3) freshness; (4) nature; (5) unstoppable energy; (6) feminist agendas; (7) use of clean language; and (8) good science. There were observed shifts in how the ads approached menstruation in each thematic area throughout the decades.

Hiding, Silencing, and Shame

Hiding, silencing, and shame are among the main negative perceptions surrounding menstruation in various cultures,[27,38] and they are prevalent in menstrual product advertisements. Menstruation is often portrayed as a hygienic crisis that needs to be managed carefully with the promoted products.[41] Commercials for menstrual products contribute to and perpetuate the notions of hiding, silencing, and shame surrounding menstruation.

First, the advertisements constantly highlight the need to keep menstrual products hidden. This concealment manifests mainly in advertisements for tampons, where the various advantages of the tampon, small and compact, are compared to pads, large and clumsy. Second, the hiding of menstrual blood is referenced, and there is no use of the word menstruation. To demonstrate the high absorbency of the products, tampons are inserted into blue-colored water or blue liquid is dripped onto pads. This visually removes the link to red blood in favor of more palatable blue fluid. The products themselves are packaged such that it is unclear what they are, so if a woman is "caught" with the product, her situation will not be discovered.

The enforced concealment of menstruation and the products point to the perception of female sexuality as something that is bound to remain hidden from view. The construction of female sexuality has been rooted in Western society for many years; therefore, "success" for women is considered to be the ability to look sexually attractive to men. Because menstruation supposedly impairs attractiveness, it is essential to hide it. Indeed, in the eyes of many men, menstruation is considered a problematic, repulsive, and disgusting phenomenon.

Safety and Security

Many menstrual product advertisements talk about the need for protection against leaks, spots, mistakes, and accidents related to menstrual blood. In a society where being caught menstruating is considered very embarrassing, this point is significant, and advertisers use it extensively in marketing strategies. Security means assurance that leaks and stains will not appear. Security is guaranteed through advertisements to sell products and provide release from the restrictions and concerns associated with menstruation. However, the dangers from which the product protects remain a mystery, and there is no direct mention of the leak against which it protects.

An argument often made in advertisements is that "hygiene" products can keep the "female secret." Protecting and maintaining the female secret is one system that helps women act as if they are not menstruating. This reflects another theme in which the ideal woman appears in public and manages to keep her menstruation a secret from everyone around her. The portrayal of this behavior as a success implies that revealing her female secret to others means she no longer represents the ideal woman and that menstruation may cause women to deviate from the expectations and limits of normal society.[56] Emphasizing the ability of the products to eliminate leaks helps promote the message that a menstrual day is no different from any other day. With the use of the products, the menstruating woman can forget about her condition and make others believe in her cleanliness. By focusing on providing security for the woman, the advertisements purport the danger involved in menstruation.

Advertisements also demonstrate how bodily secretions stain a woman and construct her as a threat to the social order. The message is that women need protection from their bodies, as do those around them. In this context, the advertisements emphasize the idea that managing the menstrual cycle is necessary every day, every month. The advertisements suggest that by using the products every month, women will never be caught. The names of the products themselves imply that menstruation should always be managed (Always, Alldays) and that the products will relieve women of their worries (Carefree). In this way, advertisers sell unnecessary products. It seems that the only way to protect the female body from itself is to accept the fact that female hygiene involves managing the menstrual cycle.

Freshness

Women are presented as naturally contaminated, and more so than men. Through the marketing and sale of menstrual products that emphasize the necessity of a disinfected, fresh, and perfumed body, women are compelled to hide the biological function of their body and menstruation. The advertisements define the femininity scale and delimit the permissible ideal: An odorless body, whose secretions are adequately treated, ensures a satisfying and happy life. Using a scent implies that menstruation is a dirty and unclean condition, and to "help" with this, manufacturers offer a variety of odor-absorbing products. The advertisements indicate that women would not need odor-absorbing products if their regulated body had no unpleasant odors or uncleanliness.

Advertisements for menstrual products contain little information about menstruation, but they provide a lot of information about the female body. The advertisements imply that a woman is not clean, although this is not explicitly stated. These messages may increase feelings of insecurity regarding the female body, especially among adolescent girls. The advertisements emphasize that a woman does not control her body and needs outside help. In addition, advertisements emphasize that a woman should always be clean and fresh. Freshness will help a woman achieve cleanliness, but more than that it will help her avoid revealing her menstrual condition. The message is that a woman will not reach an ideal state of cleanliness and freshness in the absence of these specific hygiene products due to her menstruating body.

Nature

The male–female dualism, rooted in patriarchal thought, portrays the woman as being close to nature. One reason is menstruation, which is part of the menstrual cycle and linked to the lunar cycle.[57] The use of nature in advertisements for menstrual products is thus unsurprising. The use of motifs taken from nature in advertisements for menstrual products is especially noticeable in the context of the technological age in which they were developed, because modern products would not have been developed without science and technology. Advertisements for menstrual products try to reconcile the tension between the products, which are the result of cultural and technological progress, and nature, which controls the body and its secretions. This tension is a result of the perception of dualism in hegemonic Western culture. This perception, which links femininity to body and nature and links masculinity to intellect and culture, evaluates the aspects associated with femininity in a negative manner. The man is considered the human standard, against which the female body and essence are perceived as a deviation from the norm. The female body is controlled and guided mainly by emotions, unlike the male body, which is self-controlled and rational.[58] Identifying the woman with the body and nature, and the man with intellect and culture is emblematic of the system of dualism that creates, structures, and justifies the vitality of control of superior groups over inferior groups.[14]

The use of motifs taken from nature embodies a paradox; it is precisely artificial products that must be used to return to nature. In this struggle between culture and nature, the trend of "returning to nature" to manage the body represents the domination of culture over nature. Moreover, although the advertisements promise that nature can be acquired by purchasing menstrual products,[42] to achieve this the woman must make every effort to cover and hide natural expressions of the body, such as menstruation.

Unstoppable Energy

Established brands like Kotex, Tampax, and Bodyform have been reinventing and modernizing their marketing strategies since the 1920s. Gradual changes in advertising have occurred throughout the years, but it seems that a significant change happened in the second decade of the twenty-first century. Today, most new menstrual product campaigns revolve around the concept of "breaking taboos."[59] The advertisements portray healthy and active women, thus suggesting a positive view of menstruation instead of depicting it as problematic and restrictive.[60] However, upon closer inspection, the advertisements reveal that the only way to "ensure security" is to be in line with standard social rules that require the use of these products. The modern woman can be active and attractive, not because the taboo around menstruation does not exist but because using the "right" product will ensure confidentiality and cleanliness.[41,53,61]

Advertisements often try to dispel myths about menstruation (e.g., by showing women taking part in gymnastics or swimming while menstruating), and women are often portrayed as participating in their everyday activities thanks to the freedom afforded by the products. In addition, advertisements teach women not to reveal their menstruating state and emphasize that they must act normally, continue their routine, and participate in various activities. In this context, lack of participation becomes a sign of a menstruating body. According to the advertisements, the ideal woman is active and free from bleeding.[62]

One example is Bodyform's award-winning campaign Blood Normal, which was the first to feature blood as a red liquid, purposefully chosen by the brand.[63] In the advertisement, the presentation of red blood was a seemingly provocative decision, but the blood presented was the result of injury and not menstruation (i.e., its source, physiological functions, and purposes are very different). Menstrual blood, unlike blood revealed through injury, remained shameful and hidden. Menstruation is presented as an obstacle to overcome, and the women who use the menstrual products are shown to be active, strong, safe, and in control of their lives.

Feminist Agendas

Advertisers market DMPs in alignment with the ideas of feminism and "menstrual liberation."[3,6] These ads embrace, appropriate, use, and present feminist messages. However, they also presume that women are identical, and the women shown are athletic and shapely and have the ideal physical appearance. In addition, the advertisements are ambivalent, presenting feminist and patriarchal messages together. On the one hand, the ads show that a woman can manage her life without interruption despite the many difficulties associated with menstruation, giving her control and choice. On the other hand, this liberation relies on the products. The woman must obey advertisers to free herself, so liberation is not something she can achieve on her own.

This wave of "feminist" advertisements seems to address the modern perception that previous advertisements for menstrual products are outdated and ridiculous. According to Liu and colleagues,[43] this type of advertisement represents a departure from an emphasis on femininity to more inclusive content that portrays menstruation as natural and empowering, and today's consumers are responding positively to the shift towards more progressive and diverse ads that reflect current social movements. However, despite this apparent progress, menstrual product advertisers are still driven by the perception of menstruation as disruptive and hostile, and they continue to represent it as something that must be eliminated or even discontinued. They encourage women to purchase DMPs while exploiting feminism to appeal to a more contemporary audience. This is an example of how capitalism embraces and co-opts feminism in depictions of menstruation.[64]

Since 2014, the menstrual product brand Always and its #LikeAGirl campaign have made headlines for being at the forefront of menstrual liberation, championing female empowerment and gender equality.[3] The campaign repositions the brand as advocating for gender equality and widening outdated, rigid definitions of girlhood. Women are no longer confined to typically feminine roles; instead, they are pictured playing rugby and weightlifting.[65] Although Always uses feminist agendas, there is no evidence that the company works to promote social messages in its organization or beyond its advertisements. Moreover, the company's social goals are selective: It ignores the environment while continuing to market disposable products that contribute to increased waste generation. The campaign is an example of commodity activism, whereby advertising companies use their brands and advertisement opportunities to superficially promote social activism.[66] In this context, the Always campaign uses feminist agendas to encourage the purchase of products and thus increase the company's profits.

Use of Clean Language

Menstruation is a subject that is usually not considered polite to talk about or mention. For example, the word "period" is the most popular term used to refer to this subject, indicating the generality of the process of which menstruation is only a part, and with no specific reference to the bleeding itself. Commercials often use euphemisms to describe menstruation and menstrual products. In this context, the language used in advertisements is era dependent. The word "period" was not said on-screen until 1985 in a Tampax ad.[67] This advertisement was unusual, and shocking compared to the ads that aired during that time, and it took many years for other words such as "menstruation" and "vagina" to be used.

Most advertisements do not use the word "menstruation," reinforcing the negative perceptions of menstruation and especially the embarrassment, hiding, and silencing around the subject. So, the advertisements contain minimal mention of how the products work, the associated body areas, and the genitals into which they are inserted. In the HelloFlo commercials, direct language is used, including the terms "menstruation," "menstrual cycle," and "vagina." The advertisement tries to prove the company's positive attitude towards menstruation, both in direct language and by presenting motifs representing menstrual blood. Menarche is the first menstruation, and this is presented as a milestone that represents adolescence; the girls in the advertisements long for menarche to come. However, at the same time, by celebrating the menarche as a part of "the first moon party," a link is made between the female body and nature, and, as mentioned earlier, this presentation of women as being closer to nature is responsible for the perception of women as less valuable.[57]

Good Science

In the process of medicalization of the female body and menstruation, advertisements often present an "expert" whose purpose is to authoritatively confirm the necessity of the product.[11] The advertisements use scientific knowledge, medical claims, and the approval of a professional to confirm the uniqueness of the advertised product and present its advantages over other products. The advertisements emphasize softness, comfort, innovative design, "wings," and absorption.

In 2020, Tampax created a line of ads on its YouTube channel with the comedian Amy Schumer called "Amy Visits the Gyno."[68] In these ads, Schumer is seen asking a gynecologist about menstruation and the female body. The ads attempt to refute myths about virginity and the female body, such as the loss of virginity from putting in a tampon, sleeping with a tampon in, toxic shock syndrome, etc. The gynecologist answers the questions in an informative way. Still, the questions and their answers confirm the necessity of the tampon and emphasize its advantages. Some questions specifically refer to Tampax's products. Although, on the surface, these advertisements address frequently asked questions about menstruation, they contain many tampon- and Tampax-specific questions. When addressing the ingredients of the product, the gynecologist denies that they are made from dioxide, pesticides, bleach, and gluten, but the Tampax (n.d.) website reveals ingredients that are not addressed in the ad, such as paraffin, ethoxylated fatty acid esters, PEG-100 stearate, and titanium dioxide.

Conclusions

The analysis reveals that advertisements still inherit the prevalent perceptions about menstruation; use motifs that refer to women, the female body, and nature as other; and encourage the purchase of disposable products. The identified themes reveal changes in the messages presented in advertisements throughout the years, but one main idea remains: The woman's construction as other. In this context, the advertisements' continuous strengthening of the dichotomous separation, exemplified by ecofeminist theory, influences women's consumer behavior and alienates them from their bodies.

The representation of the menstrual woman as other and menstruation suppression, as shown in the advertisements, plays a tactical role in conserving the power of capitalist consumer culture. Consumer culture relies on the excessive production and consumption of disposable products. In this way, the capitalist mechanism around menstruation encourages the constant purchase of products to be later thrown in the trash. Advertising companies have a clear interest in menstrual suppression. They take advantage of the negative perception of menstruation to encourage the purchase of disposable products that cause lasting pollution (tampons and disposable pads), even though there are ecological, cheaper, and healthier alternatives (menstrual cups and reusable pads).

An ecofeminist reading illuminates the devastating results of marketing, purchasing, and using disposable products; products that contribute to environmental damage, pollution, and waste while eliminating menstrual blood. The themes found here reflect the perception that during menstruation there is a danger of leakage of "femininity." The idea that menstruation causes women to deviate from sociocultural norms is highlighted by the product's ability to make menstrual days the same as any other day. The advertisements teach women to exercise caution, pretend that they are not menstruating, and make others believe this too. In this context, advertisements function as a tool for the external control of women. The advertisements call on women to control their bodies and menstruation by purchasing and using DMPs. Using a disposable product is portrayed as the only way to ensure that a menstruating woman can keep menstrual blood out of her body and mind.

Analyzing the hidden messages in advertisements reveals that the female body is presented negatively—as inferior, dirty, and smelly. It must be constantly regulated to conform to beauty ideals—clean, dry, fragrant, and fresh. Women internalize these messages and employ them on their bodies; they embody the notion that their bodies are less valuable when menstruating and a source of embarrassment and shame. This negative representation influences women's self-perception and causes them to adopt internal control over their external appearance and bodily fluids. In this way, the advertisements also function as a tool for internal self-control of women. To avoid contact with menstruation and keep it away from the body and mind, women turn to purchasing and using DMPs that allow them to ignore menstruation almost wholly. Following the use of DMPs, women adopt the notion that their body is inferior and a source of embarrassment and shame.[69] By using these disposable products, women willingly become the other. As a result, they move away from and suppress their bodies.

These representations of menstruation in advertisements and their effects on society also affect menstrual health. The directive to avoid contact with menstruation (physically and mentally) encourages the use of DMPs. The use of disposable products leads to a lack of awareness of the menstrual body, and the products affect the blood's color, smell, and even flow, making it harder to know if there are any problems. In addition, as a result of treating the menstrual cycle as a health disorder, the discussion surrounding it is often held only in medical terms and can only be addressed with medical solutions. Educational, sexual, and reproductive health programs are lacking, which is ultimately caused by the taboo around this subject and the view that the only "acceptable" way of addressing menstruation is through a medical approach. Achieving good menstrual health is not only a matter of ensuring access to menstrual products but also relies on individuals having the resources they need to participate fully in all spheres of life during their menstrual cycle. Menstrual health should be prioritized as an integral part of sexual and reproductive health programs, and holistic approaches to menstrual health are needed.

This chapter illuminates how the prevailing perception of menstruation structures the female body as other through disposable menstrual product advertisements. It reveals how ecofeminist theory can offer an alternative perspective to the main themes in ads that both enhance the taboo about menstruation, leading to the purchase and use of disposable products, and portray nature as inferior, ultimately reinforcing the inferiority of women to men. In this manner, ecofeminist thinking can reduce the consumption of disposable products and increase the use of reusable products, an action that might have positive benefits for women, menstruators and their bodies, and the environment.

Notes

1 Feminine Hygiene—Worldwide. statista. www.statista.com/outlook/cmo/tissue-hygiene-paper/feminine-hygiene/worldwide.
2 Peberdy E, Jones A, Green D. A Study into Public Awareness of the Environmental Impact of Menstrual Products and Product Choice. *Sustainability.* 2019; 11(2): 473. doi:https://doi.org/10.3390/su11020473.
3 Campbell R, Freeman O, Gannon V. From Overt Threat to Invisible Presence: Discursive Shifts in Representations of Gender in Menstrual Product Advertising. *Journal of Marketing Management.* 2021; 37(3–4): 216–237. doi:10.1080/02672 57X.2021.1876752.
4 Kissling EA. *Capitalizing on the Curse The Business of Menstruation.* Lynne Rienner Publishers; 2006. Accessed July 14, 2021. www.rienner.com/title/Capitalizing_on_the_Curse_The_Business_of_Menstruation.
5 McKenzie M, Bugden M, Webster A, Barr M. Advertising (In) Equality: The Impacts of Sexist Advertising on Women's Health and Wellbeing. *Women's Health Issues Paper.* (14). doi:informit.135672368547541.
6 Przybylo E, Fahs B. Empowered Bleeders and Cranky Menstruators: Menstrual Positivity and the "Liberated" Era of New Menstrual Product Advertisements. In: Bobel C, Winkler IT, Fahs B, Hasson KA, Kissling EA, Roberts TA, Eds. *The Palgrave Handbook of Critical Menstruation Studies.* Springer Singapore; 2020: 375–394. doi:10.1007/978-981-15-0614-7_30.
7 Angier N. *Woman: An Intimate Geography.* Random House; 1999. Accessed September 9, 2021. www.amazon.com/Woman-Natalie-Angier/dp/0544228103.
8 Laws S, Campling J (Eds.). *Issues of Blood: The Politics of Menstruation.* Macmillan; 1990. Accessed September 9, 2021. www.palgrave.com/gp/book/9780333482346.
9 Mead M. *Male and Female.* Penguin Books; 1950. Accessed September 9, 2021. www.abebooks.co.uk/book-search/title/male-female/author/mead/.
10 Martin E. *The Woman in the Body: A Cultural Analysis of Reproduction.* Beacon Press; 2001.
11 Shuttleworth S. Female Circulation: Medical Discourse and Popular Advertising in the Mid-Victorian Era. *Body/Politics: Women and the Discourse of Science.* Routledge; 1989; 3: 47–68.
12 Oudshoorn N. On Bodies, Technologies, and Feminisms. In: *Twentieth Century Science, Technology, and Medicine.* University of Chicago Press; 2001: 199–213.
13 Dobscha S, Ozanne JL. An Ecofeminist Analysis of Environmentally Sensitive Women Using Qualitative Methodology: The Emancipatory Potential of an Ecological Life. *Journal of Public Policy & Marketing.* 2001; 20(2): 201–214. doi:10.1509/jppm.20.2.201.17360.
14 Plumwood V. *Feminism and the Mastery of Nature.* Routledge; 1993.
15 Shiva V. *Staying Alive: Women, Ecology, and Survival in India.* Kali for Women; 1988.
16 Warren KJ. The Power and the Promise of Ecological Feminism. *Environmental Ethics.* 1990; 12(2): 125–146.

17 Warren KJ. *Ecofeminist Philosophy: A Western Perspective on What It Is and Why It Matters*. Rowman & Littlefield; 2000.

18 Robbins BD. The Objectification of Women and Nature. In: *The Medicalized Body and Anesthetic Culture*. Palgrave Macmillan; 2018: 167–180.

19 Bobel C, Kissling EA. Menstruation Matters: Introduction to Representations of the Menstrual Cycle. *Women's Studies*. 2011; 40(2): 121–126. doi:10.1080/00497878. 2011.537981.

20 Buckley T, Gottlieb A. *Blood Magic: The Anthropology of Menstruation*. University of California Press; 1988. doi:10.1525/9780520340565.

21 Roberts TA, Goldenberg J, Power C, Pyszczynski T. "Feminine Protection": The Effects of Menstruation on Attitudes Towards Women. *Psychology of Women Quarterly*. 2002; 26: 131–139. doi:10.1111/1471-6402.00051.

22 Burrows A, Johnson S. Girls' Experiences of Menarche and Menstruation. *Journal of Reproductive & Infant Psychology*. 2005; 23(3): 235–249. doi:10.1080/ 02646830500165846.

23 Fahs B. There Will Be Blood: Women's Positive and Negative Experiences with Menstruation. *Women's Reproductive Health*. 2020; 7(1): 1–16. doi:10.1080/232936 91.2019.1690309.

24 Schooler D, Ward LM, Merriwether A, Caruthers AS. Cycles of Shame: Menstrual Shame, Body Shame, and Sexual Decision-making. *Journal of Sex Research*. 2005; 42(4): 324–334. doi:10.1080/00224490509552288.

25 Fingerson L. *Girls in Power: Gender, Body, and Menstruation in Adolescence*. State University of New York Press; 2006.

26 Jackson TE, Falmagne RJ. Women Wearing White: Discourses of Menstruation and the Experience of Menarche. *Feminism & Psychology*. 2013; 23(3): 379–398. doi:10.1177/0959353512473812.

27 Chrisler JC, Marván ML, Gorman JA, Rossini M. Body Appreciation and Attitudes Toward Menstruation. *Body Image*. 2015; 12: 78–81. doi:10.1016/j.bodyim.2014. 10.003.

28 Johnston-Robledo I, Chrisler JC. The Menstrual Mark: Menstruation as Social Stigma. *Sex Roles*. 2013; 68(1–2): 9–18. doi:10.1007/s11199-011-0052-z.

29 Kowalski RM, Chapple T. The Social Stigma of Menstruation: Fact or Fiction? *Psychology of Women Quarterly*. 2000; 24(1): 74–80. doi:10.1111/j.1471-6402. 2000.tb01023.x.

30 Koff E, Rierdan J, Jacobson S. The Personal and Interpersonal Significance of Menarche. *Journal of the American Academy of Child Psychiatry*. 1981; 20(1): 148–158. doi:10.1016/s0002-7138(09)60724-x.

31 Owen L. Researching the Researchers: The Impact of Menstrual Stigma on the Study of Menstruation. *Open Library of Humanities*. 2022; 8. doi:10.16995/olh.6338.

32 Babbar K, Martin J, Ruiz J, Parray AA, Sommer M. Menstrual Health is a Public Health and Human Rights Issue. *The Lancet Public Health*. 2021; 0(0). doi:10.1016/ S2468-2667(21)00212-7.

33 Critchley HOD, Babayev E, Bulun SE, et al. Menstruation: Science and Society. *American Journal of Obstetrics and Gynecology*. 2020; 223(5): 624–664. doi:10.1016/ j.ajog.2020.06.004.

34 Holst AS, Jacques-Aviñó C, Berenguera A, et al. Experiences of Menstrual Inequity and Menstrual Health among Women and People Who Menstruate in the Barcelona Area (Spain): A Qualitative Study. *Reproductive Health*. 2022; 19(1): 45. doi:10.1186/s12978-022-01354-5.

35 Wood JM. (In)Visible Bleeding: The Menstrual Concealment Imperative. In: Bobel C, Winkler IT, Fahs B, Hasson KA, Kissling EA, Roberts TA, Eds. *The Palgrave Handbook of Critical Menstruation Studies*. Springer; 2020: 319–336. doi:10.1007/ 978-981-15-0614-7_25.

36 Henry C, Ekeroma A, Filoche S. Barriers to Seeking Consultation for Abnormal Uterine Bleeding: Systematic Review of Qualitative Research. *BMC Women's Health.* 2020; 20(1): 123. doi:10.1186/s12905-020-00986-8.

37 Andrist LC. The Implications of Objectification Theory for Women's Health: Menstrual Suppression and "Maternal Request" Cesarean Delivery. *Health Care for Women International.* 2008; 29(5): 551–565. doi:10.1080/07399330801949616.

38 Simes R, Berg M. Surreptitious Learning: Menarche and Menstrual Product Advertisements. *Health Care for Women International.* 2001; 22(5): 455–469. doi:10.1080/073993301317094281.

39 Mandziuk RM. "Ending Women's Greatest Hygienic Mistake": Modernity and the Mortification of Menstruation in Kotex Advertising, 1921–1926. *Women's Studies Quarterly.* 2010; 38(3/4): 42–62. Accessed July 14, 2021. www.jstor.org/stable/20799363.

40 Bobel C. *The Managed Body: Developing Girls and Menstrual Health in the Global South.* Springer International Publishing; 2019. doi:10.1007/978-3-319-89414-0.

41 Erchull MJ. Distancing Through Objectification? Depictions of Women's Bodies in Menstrual Product Advertisements. *Sex Roles.* 2013; 68(1–2): 32–40. doi:10.1007/s11199- 011-0004-7.

42 Kama A, Barak-Brandes S. Taming the Shame: Policing Excretions and Body Fluids in Advertisements for Hygiene Products. *European Journal of Cultural Studies.* 2013; 16(5): 582–597. doi:10.1177/1367549413491719.

43 Liu D, Schmitt M, Nowara A, Magno C, Ortiz R, Sommer M. The Evolving Landscape of Menstrual Product Advertisements in the United States: 2008–2018. *Health Care for Women International.* 2021; 0(0): 1–28. doi:10.1080/07399332.2021.1884251.

44 Dowling GR. Corporate Reputations: Should You Compete on Yours? *California Management Review.* 2004; 46(3): 19–36. doi:10.2307/41166219.

45 McDonagh P, Prothero A. Leap-frog Marketing: The Contribution of Ecofeminist Thought to the World of Patriarchal Marketing. *Marketing Intelligence & Planning.* 1997; 15(7): 361–368. doi:10.1108/02634509710193190.

46 Milne JM, Barnack-Tavlaris JL. A Comparison of the Menstrual Cup and the Intrauterine Device: Attitudes and Future Intentions. *Women's Reproductive Health.* 2019; 6(4): 271–288. doi:10.1080/23293691.2019.1653576.

47 AHPMA. Tampon Code of Practice. Published 2019. Accessed November 29, 2021. www.ahpma.co.uk/tampon_code_of_practice/.

48 Rep. Maloney CB [D N 12. H.R.1708—114th Congress (2015–2016): Robin Danielson Feminine Hygiene Product Safety Act of 2015. Published March 27, 2015. Accessed April 28, 2023. www.congress.gov/.

49 Rep. Maloney CB [D N 14. H.R.890—106th Congress (1999–2000): Tampon Safety and Research Act of 1999. Published June 23, 1999. Accessed April 28, 2023. www.congress.gov/.

50 Stewart K, Greer R, Powell M. Women's Experience of Using the Mooncup. *Journal of Obstetrics and Gynaecology.* 2010; 30(3): 285–287. doi:10.3109/01443610903572117.

51 Tu JC, Lo TY, Lai YT. Women's Cognition and Attitude with Eco-friendly Menstrual Products by Consumer Lifestyle. *International Journal of Environmental Research and Public Health.* 2021; 18(11): 5534. doi:10.3390/ijerph18115534.

52 Reame NK. Toxic Shock Syndrome and Tampons: The Birth of a Movement and a Research "Vagenda." In: Bobel C, Winkler IT, Fahs B, Hasson KA, Kissling EA, Roberts TA, Eds. *The Palgrave Handbook of Critical Menstruation Studies.* Palgrave Macmillan; 2020. Accessed April 28, 2023. www.ncbi.nlm.nih.gov/books/NBK565591/.

53 Del Saz-Rubio MM, Pennock-Speck B. Constructing Female Identities Through Feminine Hygiene TV Commercials. *Journal of Pragmatics.* 2009; 41(12): 2535–2556. doi:10.1016/j.pragma.2009.04.005.

54 Braun V, Clarke V. Thematic Analysis. In: *APA Handbook of Research Methods in Psychology, Vol 2: Research Designs: Quantitative, Qualitative, Neuropsychological, and Biological.* American Psychological Association; 2012: 57–71. doi:10.1037/13620-004.

55 Strauss A, Corbin J. Grounded Theory Methodology: An Overview. In: *Handbook of Qualitative Research.* Sage Publications, Inc.; 1994: 273–285.

56 Young IM. *On Female Body Experience: "Throwing like a Girl" and Other Essays.* Oxford University Press; 2005.

57 Ortner SB. Is Female to Male as Nature Is to Culture? *Feminist Studies.* 1972; 1(2): 5. doi:10.2307/3177638.

58 Cirksena K, Cuklanz L. Male is to Female As ____ Is to ____: A Guided Tour of Five Feminist Frameworks for Communication Studies. In: *Women Making Meaning: New Feminist Directions in Communication.* First Edition. Routledge; 1992: 18–25.

59 Røstvik CM. Mother Nature as Brand Strategy: Gender and Creativity in Tampax Advertising 2007–2009. *Enterprise Society.* 2020; 21(2): 413–452. doi:10.1017/eso.2019.36.

60 Agnew S, Sandretto S. A Case for Critical Literacy Analysis of the Advertising Texts of Menstruation: Responding to Missed Opportunities. *Gender and Education.* 2016; 28(4): 510–526. doi:10.1080/09540253.2015.1114073.

61 Luck E. Commodity Feminism and Its Body: The Appropriation and Capitalization of Body Positivity through Advertising. *Liberated Arts: A Journal for Undergraduate Research.* 2016; 2(1): 10.

62 Sitar P. Female Trouble: Menstrual Hygiene, Shame and Socialism. *Journal of Gender Studies.* 2018; 27(7): 771–787. doi:10.1080/09589236.2017.1304860.

63 *Blood Normal*; 2017. Accessed January 14, 2022. www.youtube.com/watch?v=QdW6IRsuXaQ.

64 Fraser N. Feminism, Capitalism and the Cunning of History. Published 2009.

65 *Always #LikeAGirl*; 2014. Accessed January 14, 2022. www.youtube.com/watch?v=XjJQBjWYDTs.

66 Brønn PS, Vrioni AB. Corporate Social Responsibility and Cause-related Marketing: An Overview. *null.* 2001; 20(2): 207–222. doi:10.1080/02650487.2001.11104887.

67 *Courtney Cox 1985 Tampax Commercial*; 2013. Accessed January 14, 2022. www.youtube.com/watch?v=kOHCtQfFn7E.

68 Gyno Visit Q&A | *Time to Tampax with Amy Schumer and Girlology*; 2020. Accessed January 14, 2022. www.youtube.com/watch?v=DXgmShDwopc.

69 Lamont JM, Wagner KM, Incorvati CG. The Relationship of Self-objectification and Body Shame to Attitudes Toward and Willingness to Use Reusable Menstrual Products. *Women's Reproductive Health.* 2019; 6(1): 1–16. doi:10.1080/23293691.2018.1556428.

6

HOT AND BOTHERED BY THE MENOPAUSE INDUSTRY

Mary Hunter

Long before estrogen pills were manufactured, women experienced bothersome symptoms during the menopause transition. The word *menopause* only became part of medical discourse when chemicals with certain properties were identified, synthesized, and named "hormones."[1] In creating a market for "hormone replacement therapy (HRT)," pharmaceutical manufacturers redefined healthcare for older women in the United States (US) and other high-income countries. A narrative explaining how that happened is provided below; however, how "hormone replacement therapy" is marketed is the main focus of this chapter.

Physicians were the initial marketing targets for HRT in the 1960s, and marketing menopausal hormone therapy (HT), a term preferred by academics, to physicians and other providers is still common.[2] In the twenty-first century, however, direct marketing of HT to women, particularly on the Internet, is a particularly impactful strategy. On websites and in magazines and books, HT is routinely promoted as an anti-aging and disease-prevention drug.

Most information about menopause in professional journals and popular media proclaims that symptoms women experience during and after "the midlife transition" are evidence of pathology. "Ovarian failure" is a term that signifies menopause and female aging in this discourse, and claims are made that it (menopause, AKA "ovarian failure") causes common diseases such as dementia. The marketing message is that women will suffer needlessly, and their bodies will deteriorate unless they use hormone "replacement" therapy. The purported validity of the marketing message is taken for granted by consumers of this literature, and some women become long-term users of HT.

On the other hand, most women worldwide, even those whose health insurance would pay for hormones to treat hot flashes and vaginal dryness, do not

DOI: 10.4324/9781003472711-7

consider menopause a medical condition and generally decline (or don't fill) prescriptions they are offered.[3] Having multiple reasons to appreciate the end of menstruation, most women consider hot flashes, associated sleep changes, and vaginal dryness part of normal aging. They do not reflexively assume that all age-related physical changes are related to estrogen levels. Women who reject the idea that menopause is a disease are better prepared to ignore marketing messages generated by the pharmaceutical industry.

The Medicalization of Aging in Women

In his book *The medicalization of society* (2007), Peter Conrad referred to those claiming that a specific human condition could (and should) be medically treated as "drivers" of medicalization.[4] He observed that pharmaceutical corporations are the primary drivers, and the introduction of a new drug to treat a newly named condition opens up opportunities for new profits.

Pharmaceutical companies promote drugs by working in concert with other actors, other drivers, who assist in medicalizing human conditions that were previously reasonably considered normal life experiences.[4] Common human conditions that have been medicalized include hyperactivity/low performance in children and adults, mild depression, social anxiety, and low sexual desire. There is a large market in the US, and other countries whose populations have similar access to healthcare and prescription medications, for drugs that can be used to treat these common conditions.

Additional drivers of medicalization include patient advocacy groups and professional organizations that influence guidelines for patient care.[4] Often, pharmaceutical corporations sponsor or otherwise lend support to these groups as well as to individuals within them. Social and political movements, including religious sects, act as drivers of medicalization and, conversely, drivers of de-medicalization. AIDS drug access activists and LGBTQ rights activists have advanced efforts to de-medicalize, de-criminalize, and normalize homosexuality in many countries.

Conrad cited the feminist movement in the US as a significant driver of resistance to the over-medicalization of women's conditions, such as the experiences of menstruation, premenstrual syndrome, childbirth, and menopause.[4] Feminist movements have not de-medicalized most women's common conditions/ experiences; however, feminist authors have contributed to thoughtful conversations regarding the legitimacy of specific targets of medical intervention.[5] Examining the reasons for, and adverse consequences of, high rates of surgical births is one example of such a conversation. Literature by feminists, including the global publication of *Our Bodies, Ourselves*, has helped reset and balance perspectives on women's health in an increasingly medicalized healthcare environment.[6]

In the introductory chapter of their edited book *Revisioning women, health, and healing*, Adele Clarke and Virginia Olesen wrote: "The biomedicalization of life itself ... is the key overarching, usually taken-for-granted, and often invisible social process" (p. 20).[5] They argued that this process has created a *medical industrial complex* that has grown into a global phenomenon, and a Western biotechnological view of medicine has led to a reduction in the availability of traditional medical practices. This trend includes the replacement of women-run clinics providing care using less technology with clinics that use more. It is apparent why Judy Norsigian, who co-wrote the Preface for our book, described (on the book cover) *Revisioning women, health, and healing* as "The perfect companion to *Our Bodies, Ourselves*."

With their book *Biomedicalization: Technoscience, health, and illness in the U.S.*, Clarke and colleagues extended the concept of biomedicalization to incorporate increasingly technoscientific advances that (1) permit greater surveillance of individual and population health and (2) increase options for medical intervention.[7] Health surveillance includes both risk assessment and management of patients at risk; examples of surveillance biotechnologies include genetic analyses and computer-enhanced imaging. Biotechnological advances for medical intervention include drugs such as tamoxifen to prevent breast cancer, and gene-targeted chemotherapeutic agents and state-of-the-art radiotherapy for the treatment of breast disease. Clarke and colleagues noted that clinics offering anti-aging therapies, for which patients usually pay out-of-pocket, comprise a particularly profitable and growing biotechnological medical specialty. Clarke referred to the gendering of biomedicalization, or the over-medicalization of women, as the fundamental assumption of *Our Bodies, Ourselves*.

A growing number of *Femtech* software and technology companies working to address women's biotechnological needs are highlighted in newsfeeds.[8] The term "Femtech" was first used by Ida Tin, who in 2013 founded the German company that makes Clue®, a period and ovulation tracking application, or app.[9] "From period to pregnancy tracking, Clue's got you covered." Similar products offer means for monitoring, testing, recording, and analyzing various measurements of women's bodies. *Femtech* products purport to help women prevent and treat incontinence, have better sex, track and manage menstrual cycle symptoms, avoid pregnancy, know exactly when to expect menopause, manage cancer treatment regimens, and collect this information using a cell phone. These products support the medicalization of women's everyday lives.

Conrad wrote that the diagnosis and treatment of menopause with menopausal hormone therapy (HT) is a quintessential example of medicalization resulting from the efforts of the pharmaceutical industry.[4] In the mid-twentieth century, the condition of being a woman who no longer had menstrual periods was pathologized by the pharmaceutical industry in much the same way that being a man who didn't always have a hard erection has more recently been pathologized. Viagra® has been promoted in a massive marketing effort by the same corporation, Pfizer, that long dominated the HT market. As with HT, marketers of Viagra® facilitated the medicalization of a common benign condition, and blockbuster sales have contributed billions to the cost of government-funded insurance for older adults.

Why am I Hot and Bothered?

What got me so riled up about the menopause industry? Numerous women in my social orbit were diagnosed with breast cancer while using HT. Their cancer diagnoses have spanned several decades, but most occurred in the 1990s and early 2000s when HT use was common. Examination of pharmacy claims databases indicates that up to 42 percent of US women used HT at that time, most taking estrogen and progesterone in combination.[10,11] My sense of alarm about these cancer diagnoses spiked after several friends told me they felt more upset about having to stop estrogen than about having to deal with breast cancer. One lamented (this is an exact quote): "Now I am going to look like other women my age!" Another talked her doctor into prescribing enough vaginal estrogen cream to smear on her face and body after he refused to write more prescriptions for estrogen pills.

Healthcare providers are targets for pharmaceutical marketing, including marketing that echoes the menopause industry discourse.[12] During the 1980s and 1990s, I received at least monthly, both at work and in my home mailbox, expensively produced literature from Wyeth Pharmaceuticals, which is now owned by Pfizer, informing me that I should be prescribing HT for all premenopausal, menopausal, and post-menopausal patients. Nearly all the women's health conferences I attended were sponsored by Wyeth, the manufacturer of Premarin®, and many of the continuing education courses I was required to take for ongoing certification were authored by physicians with close ties to Wyeth and other HT manufacturers. As a reader of feminist literature, I developed a focused interest in the topic of menopause, partly due to the overpromotion of HT. Ever more ubiquitous messages about HT benefits made me ever more skeptical. If something is too good to be true, it probably isn't … right?

After working for many years as a nurse practitioner, I decided to be trained to conduct research. An award from the US National Institutes of Health helped support my research training at the University of California San Francisco School of Nursing, which is where I obtained my first nursing degree in 1980. Going back to school to earn a PhD led to my editing this book.

A summary of my research on long-term users' beliefs about HT is followed by a concise history of the menopause industry. Overall, this chapter is a critique of corporate marketing that over-medicalizes menopause and a commentary on the medicalization of aging. I hope my arguments help balance the disproportionately high percentage of medical literature that promotes long-term HT as good medicine. I also hope that this examination of the marketing of HT serves as a useful example to others studying pharmaceutical marketing schemes that over-medicalize aging.

Study of Menopausal Hormone Therapy Decision-making

While earning a PhD in nursing, I conducted a qualitative study to explore users' perceptions of the risks and benefits of menopausal hormone therapy (HT) to learn who influences treatment decisions and to understand how that influence is exerted.[13] Data collection started with a pilot study in 2013 and interviews continued through 2018. To meet inclusion criteria, the 30 participants were required to be over age 60 and to have used systemic HT beyond the 5-year period considered relatively safe by panels of experts, such as the International Endocrine Society and the North American Menopause Society.[14,15]

Most participants had used HT for longer than 15 years, and their ages ranged from 60 to 80. Women were recruited with posters and on Internet message boards in the California Bay Area and a small city in the Rocky Mountain region. In hour-long interviews, participants were asked to talk about what they recalled feeling and thinking as they approached menopause and why they started HT. If they needed prompting, I inquired about information sources that had influenced their decisions to continue using HT, and I inquired whether they had any concerns about risk. Because most participants were storytellers, asking a clarifying question or "Can you tell me more about that?" was generally all I needed to do to keep a narrative moving along. Enthusiastic advocates for HT, many of the women told me they volunteered to be interviewed because of their positive experiences.

A major theme in analysis of interview transcripts was that estrogen gave these women a sense of control.[13,16] Many had used oral contraceptives, and some had transitioned directly from contraceptive pills to HT. They appreciated hormonal contraception for giving them control of their fertility and regulating menstrual bleeding, and it was not a mental stretch for them to believe that hormones were a reasonable way to manage any potential problems menopause might present. Hot flashes were reported to be a primary indication for starting HT. Only one participant had attempted to quit, and many stated a belief that hot flashes would recur if HT was ever discontinued. These women had received the message that HT could help them resist aging and prevent disease. Who wouldn't want that? Believing it *had* helped them resist aging and prevent disease, they feared and strongly resisted quitting. Rather than recognizing their innate attributes, most gave credit to HT for their attractiveness, mental acuity, athleticism, and vitality.

When asked about risk concerns, typical responses reflected skepticism about risk information, which was characterized as inconsistent and conflicting. Warnings that long-term use could potentially lead to cancer, cardiovascular disease, or dementia were not convincing or even concerning to these women. Disbelieving evidence that prolonged use could harm them, none had plans to quit.

It was an educated group, and several were medical professionals; they were confident in their ability to process risk information. Participants usually brought up disease prevention when I asked about risk concerns. They calculated that any potential risk from HT was balanced by disease prevention. At the close of interviews, participants were told where on the Internet they could obtain current information about the risks and benefits of HT.[17] I encouraged them to review the science and the advice of experts in the field regarding how long it is wise to use HT. This is the webpage I recommended: https://www.uptodate.com/contents/menopausal-hormone-therapy-benefits-and-risks#!

Most of these long-term users talked about the fear of being denied HT by health-maintenance organizations or individual providers. They had gone to great lengths to find providers who were willing to continue prescribing HT when they aged past 60. They were the primary drivers of prolonged use; their doctors had not urged them to continue. Taking HT, I concluded, was perhaps more a habit than a decision. As one woman, age 80, the wife of a medical doctor put it, "Taking Premarin® has just been part of my life for so long."

Risks of Long-term Systemic HT

Although HT is effective in reducing the frequency and intensity of hot flashes and relieving vaginal dryness, this relief comes at a potential cost, especially if systemic hormones (pills or patches) are used. Studies conducted primarily to determine whether HT prevents cardiovascular disease and dementia were funded by the US National Institutes of Health and the National Health Service in the United Kingdom (UK).[18,19] The Women's Health Initiative (WHI), a randomized controlled trial in the US that enrolled over 27,000 participants, found that users of HT experienced excess rates of breast cancer, blood clots, cardiovascular disease, and dementia, and these rates rose with length of use.[18,20,21,22] The Million Women Study (MWS), a prospective investigation that enrolled one in four of all UK women born between 1935 and 1950, confirmed the WHI's findings.[19,23] Notably, the MWS clarified that long-term estrogen-alone therapy increases the incidence of breast cancer, which was an issue not resolved by WHI data.

Although initial reports from the WHI and MWS were published over two decades ago, causing a dramatic decline in the prescription of HT, an ever-increasing number of hormone products are used by millions of women.[24]

Systemic HT risks are now known to include breast and ovarian cancer, heart disease, blood clots, thromboembolic stroke, gallbladder disease, dementia, and incontinence.[17,20,25,26] When HT is used for five years or less, the increased risk for any of these conditions is small. Vaginal estrogen, used as directed, is superior for treating vaginal symptoms, and the associated risk is low enough that long-term use is not discouraged by panels of experts.[26]

Systemic HT risks increase over time, which is why gynecology professional society prescribing guidelines discourage using it longer than five years or after age 60.[27] Nevertheless, at least one-third of HT prescriptions in the US are written for women over age 60 who have used it for longer than 5 years and who bear the greatest risk.[10] This alarming fact can be attributed to the aggressive promotion of HT by pharmaceutical corporations.[12]

A Short History of the Hormone Industry

Before surgical infection-control measures were employed, risky surgery to remove the uterus and ovaries was sometimes performed to manage "hysteria" and other physical and psychological maladies.[2] By the early part of the twentieth century, ovarian extracts (from the ovaries of cows or ovaries harvested from the women who underwent the surgeries mentioned in the previous sentence) were administered to treat symptoms such as hot flashes, sexual disinterest, and irritability. In that some women dosed with ovarian extracts had survived ovariectomies that yielded extracts for others, one might conclude that there was an element of economy in this practice model.

Starting in the late 1930s, chemical manufacturing companies in Canada, the US, the United Kingdom, and Germany invested in research to develop commercial hormone formulations.[1,2,28] One of the most successful of these companies was Ayerst/American Home Products (Canada), whose biochemist James Bertram Collip developed the estrogen drug Premarin®. Initially, Collip and biochemists at several other companies attempted to produce oral estrogen using human urine, but Collip found that mares' (horse) urine produced a less odorous and better-tasting pill. With this innovation, Ayerst got a head start in the HT market, and Premarin® was off and running to become the most profitable brand-name drug of the twentieth century.

Adolf Butenandt, who worked for Schering (Germany), utilized human urine as a base ingredient for a product marketed as Progynon®, then switched to mares' urine for an improved version.[1,2,28] Schering's Progynon2® initially competed with Premarin®, but Butenandt eventually succeeded in patenting two of the most-used non-animal-based estrogen compounds, estriol and ethynyl estradiol. Butenandt's patents were issued when some people in Germany were (1) threatening to take over most of the rest of the world, (2) imprisoning persons who Nazi leadership considered genetically inferior, (3) collecting biological specimens from prisoners for research, and (4) performing experiments on prisoners, some of which utilized Butenandt's estrogen compounds.

As word spread about the successful development and patenting of estriol and ethynyl estradiol by Butenandt, biochemists in England rushed to produce a competing non-animal-based oral estrogen.[1,2,28] The product that resulted from these efforts is diethylstilberstrol (DES), a non-steroidal synthetic estrogen that is inexpensive to make and very potent. DES was not patentable after the inventor, Edward Charles Dobbs, published the formula in the journal *Nature*. The fact that it was not patentable made the drug attractive to other chemical companies wishing to compete in the hormone market.

In the US, a group of drug manufacturers worked together to pressure the FDA to approve DES.[1,2,28] Dobbs suspected that DES was carcinogenic, and he did not recommend this drug, or other forms of synthetic estrogen, for treating symptoms of normal menopause (as distinct from premature menopause). Nevertheless, manufacturers of DES and other estrogens hired advertising firms to create a larger market, and by targeting healthy, middle-aged women, the hormone industry created a new conceptual model of menopause—a medical model. This was around the time that the word "menopause" was first used as a medical diagnosis.

DES was initially marketed to treat menopausal hot flashes; however, the side effect of pronounced nausea prevented its widespread use.[1,2,28] Without research to support using it to prevent miscarriage, and without any evidence of safety or efficacy, DES was FDA-approved and repurposed for use by women with threatened or prior spontaneous abortion. Prescribing it to pregnant women from 1940 to 1971 resulted in cancers and genital malformations in both female and male offspring. DES has also been used extensively in livestock feed, further exposing humans to this potent carcinogen through food sources and groundwater.[29]

Anti-aging Claims, Cancer, and Celebrity Endorsements

The development of a commercial estrogen market helped physicians grow their medical practices, and this is precisely how Premarin® was initially promoted in medical journals.[1,2,28] Later advertisements depicted menopausal women as ugly hags, torturing their families, and harassing doctors. Contrasting images showed attractive women on Premarin® dancing with their husbands, laughing with their children, and smiling at their doctors.

In the late 1960s, Ayerst (later acquired by Wyeth), a company that spent a million dollars annually on HT advertising, secretly paid Dr. Robert Wilson, a gynecologist, to write the bestselling book *Feminine forever*.[28] According to

Feminine forever, menopause is an estrogen deficiency degenerative disease that requires treatment of all older women, women who are otherwise "castrates." Wilson stated that HT prevented cancer, and he adamantly denied clear evidence that estrogen was carcinogenic.[28,30]

Feminine forever helped create a lasting discourse that successfully sold the concept and product known as "hormone replacement therapy." Wilson's efforts to pathologize and medicalize menopause contributed to a fear of menopause and aging that still pervades society in much of the world, and it promoted the compelling belief that estrogen could slow the aging process.[1,2,28,31] By conceptually relating serum estrogen levels to the value and self-esteem of women, Wilson helped cement in the American consciousness a connection between HT, health, and youthfulness. Dr. Wilson once remarked to Barbara Seaman, a principal founder of the feminist women's health movement, that his older patients on estrogen looked attractive in tennis outfits.[28] She countered by suggesting that perhaps it was the tennis.

With patients essentially serving as test subjects (since HT was not tested for safety before being approved by the FDA), Premarin® gained popularity and came to dominate the US HT market.[1,2,28] The fact that estrogen is a carcinogen became increasingly clear as HT prevalence grew and alarming numbers of women using Premarin® developed endometrial cancer.[32,33,34,35,36] Although Ayerst/Wyeth initially denied that its product caused cancer, the evidence was incontrovertible, and the company eventually responded by adding a progestin to its estrogen-only formulation to protect the lining of the uterus. This innovation allowed the company to regain the trust of Premarin® users, and sales of Premarin® and other HT products rebounded. By the end of the twentieth century, the prevalence of HT use among women aged 50 to 74 in the US was well over 30 percent based on insurance claims for filled prescriptions.[37] Premarin® consistently dominated the HT market.

Attractive women prominent in popular media have spoken in the media about how they benefited from HT.[38] Lauren Hutton, Suzanne Somers, Jane Fonda, and Oprah Winfrey are among celebrities who have endorsed HT on television and in books and magazines.[39,40,41,42] These women are presumed to embody prima facie evidence of estrogen's cosmetic efficacy and HT's contribution to health and fitness. This type of messaging appears to work well. A woman in my social circle in the 1990s brought a book by Suzanne Somers to a group luncheon and dominated the conversation with her own endorsement of HT. Sadly, some celebrities who have endorsed hormones have developed breast cancer, and some long-term users have died from it, including Suzanne Somers.[43]

Numerous studies have shown that women who believe HT helps them resist aging and prevent disease are more likely to use it.[44-52] Not surprisingly, HT users are more likely to have cosmetic procedures than are non-users, and they spend more on beauty products.[51] Contrary to popular belief, no peer-reviewed research has demonstrated that HT has anti-aging or cosmetic efficacy, and it is not recommended for the purpose of disease prevention.[53,54,55] Why do so many women believe otherwise?

Ghostwriting and Related Deceptive Marketing Tactics

The marketing of HT to providers includes frequent direct contact by drug detailers, AKA drug reps, the provision of samples for patients, authoring and sponsoring conferences and continuing education courses, and orchestrating the publication of professional journal articles and continuing education content with a promotional message.[56,57] Key players in the production of manuscripts supporting claims of HT safety and efficacy are certain physicians regarded as experts in the field of women's health. By agreeing to lend their names to "ghost-written" publications (manuscripts authored by marketing firms such as DesignWrite), these "thought leaders" lend an illusion of validity to marketing messages.

Estrogen and Skin Collagen

A notable example of ghostwriting is Mark Brincat, MD, who published a number of papers reporting research on estrogen and the skin starting in 1983.[58–64] Dr. Brincat began his career in London, and later practiced medicine, conducted research, and taught medicine in Malta. While his earlier papers were research reports, articles published later in his career reviewed the status of the "science" related to estrogen's efficacy in clinically improving the skin. He has consistently published articles favorable to the pharmaceutical industry. The library at UCSF maintains a Drug Industry Document Archive chronicling correspondence between Brincat, ghostwriting firms such as DesignWrite, and Wyeth personnel.[65] Items in the database are discovery documents related to breast cancer victims' lawsuits against Wyeth.

It is difficult to find a single medical journal article on the topic of estrogen's effect on skin that does not cite Dr. Brincat's work claiming the clinical/cosmetic utility of estrogen in improving wrinkling or increasing collagen thickness. I easily found a recent example while writing this chapter.[66]

The titles and abstracts of Brincat's research reports are misleading, and reported data are misinterpreted in the text of abstracts. Those who read no further than the abstract would be deceived. For example, Brincat published a 1987 paper reporting a study of estrogen's effect on skin collagen content that compared the effects of various estrogen doses and modes of administration.[59] Conclusions were derived from bench-level tests of punch-biopsied skin from the abdomens and thighs of post-menopausal women. The title of this widely cited paper is "Skin collagen changes in postmenopausal women receiving different regimens of estrogen therapy." The abstract text reads as follows:

Collagen is a widespread body constituent that is affected by estrogen status in women. Its decrease after menopause can be prevented and/or restored by estrogen treatment. We explored the effect of four different hormonal replacement regimens on total skin collagen content by measuring hydroxyproline in skin biopsy specimens taken from postmenopausal women. All regimens showed increases in skin collagen levels proportionate to the levels at the start of the treatment. Estrogen replacement therapy is shown to be prophylactic in women who have higher skin collagen levels and both prophylactic and therapeutic in women with lower skin collagen levels (p. 123).[59]

Details of the research printed in the body of the report are inconsistent with the abstract. The authors stated that there is an "optimum" skin collagen content ("O" collagen) that determines whether estrogen therapy increases collagen. The finding quoted below, taken from the *Discussion* section, is somewhat obfuscated by the bulk of the manuscript text.

Those women who had initially high skin collagen levels (who tended to be in the first years after menopause) had much smaller changes or no changes at all, and in some cases actually lost collagen. The "optimum" level of collagen at the start of the study, at which no change occurred ("O" collagen) was remarkably similar in all four groups ...
Both the mean "O" collagen levels of the four treatment groups and the individual values for each treatment group are remarkably similar to the thigh skin collagen level in the group of women treated by Brincat et al for two to ten years (221.12 ± 83.47, ug/mm2). This reinforces the hypothesis that there is an optimum thigh skin collagen content, and that there is a stage beyond which further hormone treatment is of no value (p. 126).[59]

Brincat's findings fail to support the utility of estrogen for increasing collagen content or reducing wrinkling in skin, and other scientists concluded that estrogen has no clinical benefit to skin or cosmetic efficacy.[17,53,54] Most of the women in my study said they believed HT makes skin look younger, and some asserted that they looked younger than women they knew who did not use estrogen.[13,16]

Disease Prevention Claims vs. Randomized Controlled Trial Results

Following the publication of concerning results from the WHI in 2002 that led to a precipitous drop in sales, discrediting those research findings and claiming unproven HT benefits became a major industry objective.[67] Strategies used to accomplish this disinformation campaign include citing biased industry-sponsored research, "cherry-picking" data while omitting important contextual information, omitting findings that contradict industry objectives, and widely publicizing preliminary findings favorable to the industry that were eventually proved to be premature and untrue. All these tactics illustrate a disregard for ethics in the practice of research and in research reporting,[67,68,69] and they contribute to consumer confusion.

Although the WHI, MWS, and other studies have shown that HT should not be used for disease prevention, using it to stay healthy is a major emphasis in menopause marketing, and it is a message that works. A primary reason for continuing HT given by the women in my study was to prevent disease, and most had received information about HT and disease prevention from their healthcare providers. Claiming HT prevents disease is an effective way to appeal to women who believe staying healthy benefits not only themselves but those around them. Staying on HT to stay healthy is perceived as consistent with being a good wife, mother, and productive member of society.

Ghostwriting has not only been used to claim unproven benefits; it has also been used to discredit research showing that long-term use of HT comes with risk. Forensic analysis of HT discourse in medical journal articles by Fugh-Burman and colleagues found that articles with a promotional tone were twice as likely to be authored by physicians with ties to hormone manufacturers than articles written by others.[56,57] They found the following themes in articles written by authors with industry ties: (1) The risks of HT have been exaggerated, (2) Randomized clinical trials are not better than observational studies for determining these risks, (3) The study populations used in the WHI were inappropriate for determining risks, (4) Ongoing studies are expected to demonstrate protective effects from HT (disease prevention), and (5) Formulations and doses have different risk/ benefit profiles, so prescriptions tailored to an individual woman based on her unique attributes may be beneficial and have minimal risk. Articles by different "thought leaders" with ties to the pharmaceutical industry that this team examined contained entire paragraphs of text repeated word-for-word. Articles authored by gynecology specialists generally minimize the risks of HT compared with articles written by other medical specialists or generalists. Gynecology specialists, much more than internists or family physicians, are targeted by hormone drug representatives.[67] Gynecology specialists also receive marketing messages through professional organizations such as the North American Menopause Society (NAMS), which was renamed The Menopause Society in 2023.

The Kronos Early Estrogen Prevention Study (KEEPS) illustrates several of the strategies outlined by Fugh-Berman and her colleagues.[70] Critics of the WHI study design argued that findings of a higher incidence of cardiovascular disease (CVD) and dementia in users was due to the initiation of HT well after menopause. The KEEPS trial tested a "timing" hypothesis that posited that HT, when started early in menopause, would provide protection from CVD and/or cognitive decline.[71,72] The aim of the study was to determine whether estrogen, when taken early in menopause, would produce clinically significant biomarkers showing evidence of protection. This study, supported by hormone manufacturers, began in 2005 and ended in 2012. KEEPS authors apparently anticipated that their data would discredit the WHI findings.

At the 2012 annual meeting of NAMS, authors of the KEEPS study announced that they had preliminary findings showing that HT was protective against CVD and cognitive decline when started early in menopause. (A NAMS webpage with the KEEPS announcement, last accessed in 2018, has since been deleted.) Press releases and related articles appeared widely in popular news outlets such as *USA Today* and *WebMD*, giving the public the impression that there was evidence to support these conclusions. However, the assertions made in 2012 were not supported by study data, and it was not until 2014 that results on CVD outcomes showing no protection were published in a peer-reviewed journal.[72] Unlike the premature and false claims made in 2012, the actual findings were not announced in press releases or displayed on the NAMS website.

KEEPS results on cognition were eventually published in 2015.[73] The authors cherry-picked data to report transient beneficial mood effects with small to medium effect sizes with oral, but not transdermal, estrogen. The KEEPS cognition findings were not widely publicized. Reanalysis of KEEPS study data published in 2019 and 2021 also failed to yield results supporting claims of disease protection. KEEPS study publications, despite unimpressive findings, provided sponsors with opportunities to editorially criticize the WHI and to reiterate the possibility that future studies would show that HT "tailored to individual women" and "started early" might be beneficial for preventing CVD or cognitive decline.[74,75]

Results of the KEEPS studies are modest and straightforward: (1) Short-term use of HT poses low risk to users, and (2) There is no evidence that HT prevents CVD or cognitive decline.[75] Nevertheless, I encountered medical professionals who believed that the KEEPS studies' results supported using HT for disease prevention long after publication of the final results.

More recent research involves brain-imaging studies that are claimed to suggest that systemic estrogen prevents the accumulation of proteins associated with Alzheimer's disease.[76-80] This is another project, like KEEPS, that incorporates the hypothesis that using systemic estrogen early in menopause can prevent disease. It is also an example of how imaging biotechnology can be employed to create a promotional narrative for HT.

Research associated with Lisa Mosconi, PhD at Weill Cornell has been widely publicized in medical "news" outlets and in numerous videos, including a TED talk.[76-80] This is third-party marketing, not peer-reviewed science.

Despite Dr. Mosconi stating that only certain women would potentially benefit, publicity about the project serves to bolster the menopause industry's characterization of HT as a disease-prevention drug. None of the women in my study appeared to appreciate cautionary details in research reports. Women who have seen Dr. Mosconi's videos will probably remember her attractiveness and sexy Italian accent, the colorful brain images, and the tantalizing suggestion that HT, when taken at just the right time, can prevent Alzheimer's disease. Moreover, women who start HT believing it can prevent Alzheimer's disease are unlikely to believe they should quit when they are no longer in "early menopause."

The North American Menopause Society/The Menopause Society

Themes identified by Fugh-Berman and colleagues[56,57] strongly resemble themes in the 2012 "Hormone Therapy Position Statement of the North American Menopause Society."[81] Several individuals on the Advisory Panel for the 2012 Position Statement reported relationships with hormone manufacturers. Subsequent revisions of the Position Statement have contained what I read to be more moderate and cautionary wording about the risks of long-term HT than earlier versions.[26,82]

For many years, the NAMS website hosted a decision tool based on the impact of menopausal symptoms on "quality of life" developed by Wulf Utian, founder of the organization.[83] The tool was supposed to help women make decisions about whether to start HT and how long to use it. (The decision tool has since been removed from The Menopause Society's website.) Regarding the process of clinical decision-making, the quality-of-life decision tool (and the catchy phrase itself) functioned as a "short circuit," in that critical examination of long-term HT risk vs. benefit was deftly circumvented as soon as a woman confirmed that quality of life was her priority. "Quality of life" was a phrase used by nearly all the participants in my study, usually while reporting their doctors' advice to balance potential risks of HT with quality of life.[13]

An ongoing strategy to persuade women to start hormone therapy early in perimenopause was bolstered by a 2013 reanalysis (manipulation) of WHI mortality data.[84,85] Predictably, this effort was associated with physicians who had ties to NAMS.[86] Published in the *Journal of the American Medical Association (JAMA)*, the research report argued that early adoption of HT prevents excess (premature) mortality. Despite subsequent publication in the *American Journal of Public Health* of a rebuttal by lead WHI researchers explaining fatal errors in the statistical methods used in the reanalysis,[87] the argument for early use of HT to prevent premature death has steadily gained traction. Citations of this article in medical literature are common, and references to the reanalysis in lay literature are even more numerous and potentially impactful.

Widespread reporting of excess mortality ostensibly attributable to the avoidance of HT is reminiscent of an earlier approach to HT promotion. Claims for disease prevention were based on observational data, and a key reason for conducting the WHI study was to prove with a randomized controlled trial that disease prevention from the use of HT was real and significant.[20] Some researchers were concerned that the study would show significant cardiovascular benefits from HT, and they feared that the study would be discontinued before breast cancer risk was determined.[3] Ironically, the study was halted early due to excess breast cancer diagnoses in the estrogen and progestin treatment group.

Both the WHI and MWS clearly showed that observational data were misleading, and that HT does, in fact, cause disease. As outlined earlier in this chapter, the hormone industry has worked diligently since 2002 to characterize WHI and MWS findings as faulty and unconvincing.[12,88] Misinterpreting WHI data to try to prove that women's lives have been cut short by not using HT is just another marketing ploy.

The reduced mortality argument may seem plausible to readers of pro-HT literature for the same reasons that HT disease prevention claims are easily believed. Confirmation bias accounts for some of this phenomenon (i.e., people believe information that confirms their existing beliefs). Users of HT are generally more socially privileged and healthy than average, and images of youthful-appearing, physically active women (who look like they will live long lives) are pictured in HT marketing materials. Dr. Wilson's patients on estrogen looked good in tennis outfits? Yes, it's probably the tennis.

NAMS has long been a vocal proponent of HT, and its education platform is ideal for promoting menopause industry products. As noted on its website, NAMS addresses the needs of patients, clinicians, and corporate sponsors.[89] As a 501c3 corporation, the organization actively solicits charitable donations from companies and individuals to be used to educate the membership and the public about menopause.[90]

The one annual meeting I attended in 2018 presented a thoroughly medicalized model of menopause, and menopause was generally catastrophized. A young woman I met at the conference, a midwife who was there to be trained to become a "NAMS-certified menopause practitioner," remarked that she previously had no idea that hot flashes were "excruciating." Displays of pharmaceutical products and medical devices filled the conference ballroom, and most continuing education (CE) offerings were sponsored by industry partners. My perception, as a decades-long reader of the NAMS journal *Menopause* and as someone who has taken CE courses sponsored by pharmaceutical corporations partnering with NAMS, is that alliances between the pharmaceutical industry and NAMS have biased the organization's educational content and its clinical guidance.

A 2010 analysis of partisan editorial perspectives in medical literature singled out the NAMS journal *Menopause* as hosting editorials that were *less* partisan than those in *Climacteric,* the International Menopause Society journal, and *Maturitas,* another international journal dealing with midlife health issues.[91] It is worth noting, however, that the editorial examples analyzed in that study were published in 2004, which was shortly after the WHI results were widely publicized in the US, a time when articles about HT reflected concerns about over-prescribing. As the pharmaceutical industry accelerated efforts to discredit the WHI, editorials in all three of these professional journals became increasingly partisan, and the content of research articles reflects this bias.

In recent years, I have observed subtle changes to the content and tone of The Menopause Society's communications, including its educational videos and *Menopause* journal articles, that may suggest some resistance to industry influence or an attempt to present a balanced perspective. Or maybe not. An opinion piece in the October 2023 issue of *Menopause* characterized WHI breast cancer findings as "misinterpreted," "misleading," and "meaningless."[92]

Conclusions

Throughout the world, differences in HT uptake reflect differences in social class, racial and ethnic identity, and place of residence; additionally, users of HT are often well-educated and health-conscious.[1,3,93] They typically have prescription drug insurance that pays for FDA-approved pills and patches sold by major pharmaceutical corporations, and most women over age 65 are on public-funded health insurance for seniors.[10,24,94] Prescription drug insurance generally covers HT for postmenopausal women of any age, so long as the prescriber uses the correct diagnosis code for hot flashes. The code label, formerly worded "vasomotor symptoms," now reads "menopausal and other perimenopausal disorders." Most HT users can afford to pay out-of-pocket for compounded hormones, which may be used instead of, or in addition to, FDA-approved products. Several participants in my study used a combination of compounded and FDA-approved HT, paying out-of-pocket for compounded hormones and for office visits to consultants facilitating access to them.[13,16] This strategy was a last resort when medical doctors or nurse practitioners refused to prescribe exactly what the patient requested.

Survey data in the US suggest that sales of non-FDA-approved HT (i.e., compounded hormones) are roughly equal to sales of FDA-approved pills and patches sold by major pharmaceutical corporations.[24] Accurate counts of women using compounded HT are unknown because there is no practical way to track sales. US National Ambulatory Medical Care Survey data indicate that approximately 4 percent of US women over age 65 use FDA-approved HT;[95] however, combined with the use of compounded hormones, the prevalence of HT is considerably higher.

Ubiquitous Internet promotion of hormones claiming anti-aging efficacy partially explains the persistent demand for products in both FDA-approved and compounded HT categories. Manufacturers of the basic chemical constituents used in most formulations supply them in bulk to the manufacturers of both types of HT. I sense that a sustained and heated controversy about which category of HT works better and is safer serves to accelerate sales and ensure the profitability of the entire menopause industry. Pfizer and other pharmaceutical corporations no longer need to factor payment for damages into earnings projections, because black box warnings and limited liability protect them from lawsuits. It's a win-win situation for these corporations.

Most women who are prescribed HT live in countries where pharmaceutical companies focus marketing efforts. In 2022 alone, the global hormone therapy market was valued at over $21 billion (US), with a 6.6 percent predicted annual rate of growth.[96] Although this figure includes forms of hormone therapy other than estrogen and progesterone (i.e., testosterone, human growth hormone, and thyroid hormones), menopausal HT comprises 44 percent of the total. The US accounts for at least 40 percent of the total global HT market. Other countries with large markets for HT include Canada, UK, Germany, France, Italy, Spain, Denmark, Sweden, Norway, Japan, China, India, Australia, South Korea, Thailand, Brazil, Mexico, Argentina, South Africa, Saudi Arabia, the United Arab Emirates, and Kuwait.

Maximizing the numbers of filled prescriptions for women convinced that hormones help them stay youthful and healthy is clearly the primary objective of this industry. To sell as many pills, patches, and creams as possible, multinational pharmaceutical corporations strive to convince prescribers and their patients that long-term HT is not associated with a significant disease burden and professional society guidelines recommending short-term use are overly cautious.

I am *hot and bothered* by the fact that the menopause industry leverages fear to sell hormones by using false claims of anti-aging efficacy and disease prevention. Seductive and deceptive marketing messages sustain a spurious risk vs. benefit narrative about HT that belies a contempt for older women and a callous disregard for women's health. With the world's population aging rapidly, medicalizing aging to sell drugs is an increasingly common marketing practice. The successful marketing of HT suggests that the pharmaceutical industry will use similar strategies to market other "anti-aging" drugs.

Notes

1 Coney S. *The menopause industry: How the medical establishment exploits women.* Hunter House; 1994.
2 Watkins ES. *The estrogen elixir: A history of hormone replacement therapy in America.* Johns Hopkins University Press; 2007: ix.

3 Woods NF. Midlife women's health: Conflicting perspectives of health care providers and midlife women and consequences for health. In: Clarke AO, Olesen VL, Ed., *Revisioning women, health, and healing.* Routledge; 1999.

4 Conrad P. *The medicalization of society.* Johns Hopkins University Press; 2007.

5 Clarke AE, Olesen VL. *Revisioning women, health, and healing: Feminist, cultural, and technoscience perspectives.* Routledge; 1999: x.

6 Davis K. *The making of Our bodies, ourselves: How feminism travels across borders.* Next wave. Duke University Press; 2007: xii.

7 Clarke AE. *Biomedicalization: Technoscience, health, and illness in the U.S.* Duke University Press; 2010: ix.

8 Nayeri F. Is "Femtech" the next big thing in health care? *The New York Times.* April 7, 2021. Accessed 19 November, 2023. www.nytimes.com/2021/04/07/health/femtech-women-health-care.html.

9 Dodgson L. The entrepreneur who coined the term "FemTech" founded a period tracking app that's helping women understand and accept their bodies. *Business Insider.* 2020.

10 Steinkellner AR, Denison SE, Eldridge SL, Lenzi LL, Chen W, Bowlin SJ. A decade of postmenopausal hormone therapy prescribing in the United States: Long-term effects of the Women's Health Initiative. *Menopause.* June 2012; 19(6): 616–621. doi:10.1097/gme.0b013e31824bb039.

11 Hersh AL, Stefanick ML, Stafford RS. National use of postmenopausal hormone therapy: Annual trends and response to recent evidence. *Journal of the American Medical Association.* January 7, 2004; 291(1): 47–53. doi:10.1001/jama.291.1.47.

12 Fugh-Berman A. The science of marketing: How pharmaceutical companies manipulated medical discourse on menopause. *Women's Reproductive Health.* January 2, 2015; 2(1): 18–23. doi:10.1080/23293691.2015.1039448.

13 Hunter MM. Hormone therapy decision making in older women. Doctoral. University of California San Francisco. ISBN 978043876035. https://escholarship.org/uc/item/70v4k4b2.

14 Stuenkel CA, Davis SR, Gompel A, et al. Treatment of symptoms of the menopause: An Endocrine Society Clinical Practice Guideline. *Journal of Clinical Endocrinology and Metabolism.* November 2015; 100(11): 3975–4011. doi:10.1210/jc.2015-2236.

15 North American Menopause Society. The 2012 Hormone Therapy Position Statement of The North American Menopause Society. *Menopause.* March 2012; 19(3): 257–271. doi:10.1097/gme.0b013e31824b970a.

16 Hunter MM, Huang AJ, Wallhagen MI. "I'm going to stay young": Belief in anti-aging efficacy of menopausal hormone therapy drives prolonged use despite medical risks. *PloS one.* 2020; 15(5): e0233703. doi:10.1371/journal.pone.0233703.

17 Martin KB. Menopausal hormone therapy: Benefits and risks. UpToDate. Accessed January 20, 2024. www.uptodate.com/contents/menopausal-hormone-therapy-benefits-and-risks#!.

18 Manson JE, Chlebowski RT, Stefanick ML, et al. Menopausal hormone therapy and health outcomes during the intervention and extended poststopping phases of the Women's Health Initiative randomized trials. *Journal of the American Medical Association.* October 2, 2013; 310(13): 1353–1368. doi:10.1001/jama.2013.278040.

19 Beral V. Breast cancer and hormone-replacement therapy in the Million Women Study. *The Lancet.* August 9, 2003; 362(9382): 419–427.

20 Rossouw JE, Anderson GL, Prentice RL, et al. Risks and benefits of estrogen plus progestin in healthy postmenopausal women: Principal results From the Women's Health Initiative randomized controlled trial. *Journal of the American Medical Association.* July 17, 2002; 288(3): 321–333. doi:10.1001/jama.288.3.321.

21 Shumaker SA, Legault C, Kuller L, et al. Conjugated equine estrogens and incidence of probable dementia and mild cognitive impairment in postmenopausal women: Women's Health Initiative Memory Study. *Journal of the American Medical Association.* June 23, 2004; 291(24): 2947–2958. doi:10.1001/jama.291.24.2947.

22 Shumaker SA, Legault C, Rapp SR, et al. Estrogen plus progestin and the incidence of dementia and mild cognitive impairment in postmenopausal women: The Women's Health Initiative Memory Study: A randomized controlled trial. *Journal of the American Medical Association.* May 28, 2003; 289(20): 2651–2662. doi:10.1001/jama.289.20.2651.

23 Beral V, Banks E, Reeves G. Million Women Study C. Effects of estrogen-only treatment in postmenopausal women. *Journal of the American Medical Association.* August 11, 2004; 292(6): 684; author reply 685–686. doi:10.1001/jama.292.6.684-a.

24 Gass ML, Stuenkel CA, Utian WH, et al. Use of compounded hormone therapy in the United States: Report of The North American Menopause Society Survey. *Menopause.* December 2015; 22(12): 1276–1284. doi:10.1097/GME.0000000000000553.

25 Manson JE, Chlebowski RT, Stefanick ML, et al. Menopausal hormone therapy and health outcomes during the intervention and extended poststopping phases of the Women's Health Initiative Randomized Trials. *Journal of the American Medical Association.* 2013; 310(13): 1353–1368. doi:10.1001/jama.2013.278040.

26 NAMS. The 2022 Hormone Therapy Position Statement of The North American Menopause Society. *Menopause.* July 1, 2022; 29(7): 767–794. doi:10.1097/gme.0000000000002028.

27 Martin K, Barbieri R. Treatment of menopausal symptoms with hormone therapy. UpToDate.com. Updated January 21, 2024. www.uptodate.com/contents/treatment-of-menopausal-symptoms-with-hormone-therapy.

28 Seaman B. *The greatest experiment ever performed on women.* Hyperion; 2003.

29 Kolok AS, Ali JM, Rogan EG, Bartelt-Hunt SL. The fate of synthetic and endogenous hormones used in the US beef and dairy industries and the potential for human exposure. *Current Environmental Health Reports.* June 2018; 5(2): 225–232. doi:10.1007/s40572-018-0197-9.

30 The marketing of menopause: Historically, hormone therapy heavy on promotion, light on science. Accessed January 18, 2018. https://www.npr.org/2002/08/08/1148021/marketing-menopause. Radio broadcast and web page.

31 Rothman S, Rothman D. *The pursuit of perfection: The promise and perils of medical enhancement.* Random House; 2003.

32 Antunes CM, Strolley PD, Rosenshein NB, et al. Endometrial cancer and estrogen use. Report of a large case-control study. *The New England Journal of Medicine.* January 4, 1979; 300(1): 9–13. doi:10.1056/nejm197901043000103.

33 Mack TM, Pike MC, Henderson BE, et al. Estrogens and endometrial cancer in a retirement community. *The New England Journal of Medicine.* June 3, 1976; 294(23): 1262–1267. doi:10.1056/nejm197606032942304.

34 McDonald TW, Annegers JF, O'Fallon WM, Dockerty MB, Malkasian GD, Jr., Kurland LT. Exogenous estrogen and endometrial carcinoma: Case-control and incidence study. *American Journal of Obstetrics and Gynecology.* March 15, 1977; 127(6): 572–580. doi:10.1016/0002-9378(77)90351-9.

35 Smith DC, Prentice R, Thompson DJ, Herrmann WL. Association of exogenous estrogen and endometrial carcinoma. *The New England Journal of Medicine.* December 4, 1975; 293(23): 1164–1167. doi:10.1056/nejm197512042932302.

36 Ziel HK, Finkle WD. Increased risk of endometrial carcinoma among users of conjugated estrogens. *The New England Journal of Medicine.* December 4, 1975; 293(23): 1167–1170. doi:10.1056/nejm197512042932303.

37 Ettinger B, Wang SM, Leslie RS, et al. Evolution of postmenopausal hormone therapy between 2002 and 2009. *Menopause*. June 2012; 19(6): 610–615. doi:10.1097/gme.0b013e31823a3e5d.

38 Elkins C. Celebrities team with big pharma to promote drugs, disease awareness. Drug Watch. Accessed January 18, 2024. www.drugwatch.com/news/2015/11/09/celebrity-and-big-pharma-drug-promotion/.

39 Oprah.com. To: Oprah Winfrey; Subject: Hormones; What I know for sure. Oprah.com. Accessed January 18, 2024. www.oprah.com/spirit/what-oprah-knows-for-sure-about-menopause-and-hormones,

40 Kotz D. Why Suzanne Somers loves bioidentical hormones. US News and World Report. Accessed January 18, 2024. https://health.usnews.com/health-news/blogs/on-women/2009/03/25/why-suzanne-somers-loves-bioidentical-hormones.

41 Meadows S. Why is Lauren Hutton smiling? Hormones! Newsweek2000. Accessed January 18, 2024. www.newsweek.com/why-lauren-hutton-smiling-hormones-158001.

42 Cutler W. Dr. Cutler reviews Jane Fonda's book, PRIME TIME. Accessed January 18, 2024. www.athenainstitute.com/mediaarticles/janefondabook.html.

43 Liz S. Suzanne Somers pioneered the role of celebrity purveyor of medical misinformation. *Los Angeles Times*. October 19, 2023. www.latimes.com/science/story/2023-10-19/suzanne-somers-pioneered-the-role-of-celebrity-purveyor-of-medical-misinformation.

44 Fauconnier A, Ringa V, Delanoe D, Falissard B, Breart G. Use of hormone replacement therapy: Women's representations of menopause and beauty care practices. *Maturitas*. June 30, 2000; 35(3): 215–228.

45 Fisher WA, Sand M, Lewis W, Boroditsky R. Canadian menopause study-I: Understanding women's intentions to utilise hormone replacement therapy. *Maturitas*. November 30, 2000; 37(1): 1–14.

46 French LM, Smith MA, Holtrop JS, Holmes-Rovner M. Hormone therapy after the Women's Health Initiative: A qualitative study. *BMC Family Practice*. October 23, 2006; 7: 61. doi:10.1186/1471-2296-7-61.

47 Hunter MS. Predictors of menopausal symptoms: Psychosocial aspects. *Bailliere's Clinical Endocrinology and Metabolism*. January 1993; 7(1): 33–45.

48 Hunter MS, Liao KL. Intentions to use hormone replacement therapy in a community sample of 45-year-old women. *Maturitas*. November 1994; 20(1): 13–23.

49 Hunter MS, O'Dea I, Britten N. Decision-making and hormone replacement therapy: A qualitative analysis. *Social Science and Medicine*. November 1997; 45(10): 1541–1548.

50 Kolip P, Hoefling-Engels N, Schmacke N. Attitudes toward postmenopausal long-term hormone therapy. *Qualitative Health Research*. February 2009; 19(2): 207–215. doi:10.1177/1049732308328053.

51 Limouzin-Lamothe MA. What women want from hormone replacement therapy: Results of an international survey. *European Journal of Obstetrics, Gynecology, and Reproductive Biology*. April 1996; 64 Suppl: S21–24.

52 Stephens C, Budge RC, Carryer J. What is this thing called hormone replacement therapy? Discursive construction of medication in situated practice. *Qualitative Health Research*. March 2002; 12(3): 347–359. doi:10.1177/104973202129119937.

53 FDA. Menopause & hormones common questions. June 17, 2020. www.fda.gov/media/130242/download.

54 Sator PG, Sator MO, Schmidt JB, et al. A prospective, randomized, double-blind, placebo-controlled study on the influence of a hormone replacement therapy on skin aging in postmenopausal women. *Climacteric: The Journal of the International Menopause Society*. August 2007; 10(4): 320–334. doi:10.1080/13697130701444073.

55 Martin K, Barbieri R. Menopausal hormone therapy benefits and risks. Online database. UpToDate.com. Accessed January 20, 2024. https://www.uptodate.com/contents/menopausal-hormone-therapy-benefits-and-risks.

56 Fugh-Berman A, McDonald C, Bell A, Bethards E, Scialli A. Promotional tone in reviews of menopausal hormone therapy after the Women's Health Initiative: An analysis of published articles. *PLoS Medicine*. March 2011; 8(3): e1000425. doi:10.1371/journal.pmed.1000425.

57 Fugh-Berman A. The haunting of medical journals: How ghostwriting sold "HRT". *PLoS Medicine*. September 2010; 7(9): e1000335. doi:10.1371/journal.pmed.1000335.

58 Brincat M, Moniz CF, Studd JW, Darby AJ, Magos A, Cooper D. Sex hormones and skin collagen content in postmenopausal women. *British Medical Journal (Clinical Research Edition)*. November 5, 1983; 287(6402): 1337–1338.

59 Brincat M, Versi E, Moniz CF, Magos A, de Trafford J, Studd JW. Skin collagen changes in postmenopausal women receiving different regimens of estrogen therapy. *Obstetrics and Gynecology*. July 1987; 70(1): 123–127.

60 Brincat MP. Hormone replacement therapy and the skin. *Maturitas*. May 29, 2000; 35(2): 107–117. doi:10.1016/s0378-5122(00)00097-9.

61 Raine-Fenning NJ, Brincat MP, Muscat-Baron Y. Skin aging and menopause: Implications for treatment. *American Journal of Clinical Dermatology*. 2003; 4(6): 371–378. doi:10.2165/00128071-200304060-00001.

62 Brincat MP. Oestrogens and the skin. *Journal of Cosmetic Dermatology*. January 2004; 3(1): 41–49. doi:10.1111/j.1473-2130.2004.00056.x.

63 Brincat MP, Baron YM, Galea R. Estrogens and the skin. *Climacteric: The Journal of the International Menopause Society*. June 2005; 8(2): 110–123. doi:10.1080/13697130500118100.

64 Calleja-Agius J, Brincat M. The effect of menopause on the skin and other connective tissues. *Gynecological Endocrinology: The Official Journal of the International Society of Gynecological Endocrinology*. April 2012; 28(4): 273–277. doi:10.3109/09513590.2011.613970.

65 UCSF Drug Industry Documents. Brincat/Designwrite Documents. UCSF. Accessed December 12, 2023. www.industrydocuments.ucsf.edu/drug/results/#q=Brincat&h=%7B%22hideDuplicates%22%3Afalse%2C%22hideFolders%22%3Atrue%7D&subsite=drug&cache=true&count=41.

66 Zouboulis CC, Blume-Peytavi U, Kosmadaki M, et al. Skin, hair and beyond: The impact of menopause. *Climacteric: The Journal of the International Menopause Society*. October 2022; 25(5): 434–442. doi:10.1080/13697137.2022.2050206.

67 Fugh-Berman A, Scialli A. Gynecologists and estrogen: An affair of the heart. *Perspectives in Biology and Medicine*. Winter 2006; 49(1): 115–130. doi:10.1353/pbm.2006.0006.

68 Fugh-Berman A, McDonald CP, Bell AM, Bethards EC, Scialli AR. Promotional tone in reviews of menopausal hormone therapy after the Women's Health Initiative: An analysis of published articles. *PLoS Medicine*. March 2011; 8(3): e1000425. doi:10.1371/journal.pmed.1000425.

69 Fugh-Berman A, Pearson C. The overselling of hormone replacement therapy. *Pharmacotherapy*. September 2002; 22(9): 1205–1208.

70 KLRI. KEEPS Study. Kronos Longevity Research Institute. January 30, 2018. https://clinicaltrials.gov/ct2/show/NCT00154180.

71 Miller V, Taylor H, Naftolin F, Manson J, Gleason C, Brinton E., Kling J, CedarsM, Dowling N, Kantarci K, Harmon S. Lessons from KEEPS: The Kronos Early Estrogen Prevention Study. *Climacteric: The Journal of the International Menopause Society*, April 2021; 24(2): 139–145.

72 Harman SM, Brinton EA, Cedars M, et al. KEEPS: The Kronos Early Estrogen Prevention Study. *Climacteric :The Journal of the International Menopause Society.* March 2005; 8(1): 3–12. doi:10.1080/13697130500042417.

73 Gleason CE, Dowling NM, Wharton W, et al. Effects of hormone therapy on cognition and mood in recently postmenopausal women: Findings from the randomized, controlled KEEPS-Cognitive and Affective Study. *PLoS Medicine.* June 2015; 12(6): e1001833; discussion e1001833. doi:10.1371/journal.pmed.1001833.

74 Miller VM, Manson JE. Women's Health Initiative Hormone Therapy Trials: New insights on cardiovascular disease from additional years of follow up. *Current Cardiovascular Risk Reports.* June 1 2013; 7(3): 196–202. doi:10.1007/s12170-013-0305-1.

75 Miller VM, Naftolin F, Asthana S, et al. The Kronos Early Estrogen Prevention Study (KEEPS): What have we learned? *Menopause.* September 2019; 26(9): 1071–1084. doi:10.1097/gme.0000000000001326.

76 Weil Cornell Newsroom. Study suggests estrogen to prevent Alzheimer's warrants renewed research interest. Accessed December 17, 2023. https://news.weill.cornell. edu/news/2023/10/study-suggests-estrogen-to-prevent-   alzheimer%E2%80%99s-warrants-renewed-research-interest.

77 LaMotte, S. Sweet spot for HRT may reduce dementia risk by nearly a third, study says. CNN Health. November 2, 2023. www.cnn.com/2023/11/02/health/hormone-replacement-dementia-wellness/index.html.

78 Velasquez S. Dr. Lisa Mosconi's menopause brain research is reshaping the way we view hormone therapy. Sheknows. November 19, 2023. Accessed November 19, 2023. www.msn.com/en-us/health/medical/dr-lisa-mosconi-s-menopause-brain-research-is-reshaping-the-way-we-view-hormone-therapy/ar-AA1jScsh.

79 Elsesser K. Here's the current thinking on hormone therapy (It's not what you heard 20 years ago). Forbes, 2022. www.forbes.com/sites/kimelsesser/2022/04/19/heres-the-current-thinking-on-hormone-therapy-its-not-what-you-heard-20-years-ago/?sh=780c69074787.

80 How menopause affects the brain. Video accessed November 19, 2023. www.ted. com/talks/lisa_mosconi_how_menopause_affects_the_brain.

81 NAMS. The 2012 hormone therapy position statement of The North American Menopause Society. *Menopause.* March 2012; 19(3): 257–271. doi:10.1097/gme. 0b013e31824b970a.

82 NAMS. The 2017 hormone therapy position statement of The North American Menopause Society. *Menopause.* July 2017; 24(7): 728–753. doi:10.1097/GME. 0000000000000921.

83 Utian WH. Menopause QOL Instrument (UQOL). Accessed June 17, 2020. www.menopause.org/publications/clinical-practice-materials/menopause-qol-instrument-(uqol).

84 Sarrel PM, Njike VY, Vinante V, Katz DL. The mortality toll of estrogen avoidance: An analysis of excess deaths among hysterectomized women aged 50 to 59 years. *American Journal of Public Health.* September 2013; 103(9): 1583-1588. doi:10.2105/ajph.2013.301295.

85 Langer RD, Simon JA, Pines A, et al. Menopausal hormone therapy for primary prevention: Why the USPSTF is wrong. *Climacteric: The Journal of the International Menopause Society.* October 2017; 20(5): 402–413. doi:10.1080/13697137.2017. 1362156.

86 The 2017 hormone therapy position statement of The North American Menopause Society. *Menopause.* November 2018; 25(11): 1362–1387. doi:10.1097/gme. 0000000000001241.

87 Prentice RL, Manson JE, Anderson GL, et al. Women's health initiative view of estrogen avoidance and all-cause mortality. *American Journal of Public Health.* December 2013; 103(12): e2. doi:10.2105/ajph.2013.301604.

88 Fugh-Berman A, Siwek J. Compromising the medical literature: The hidden influence of industry-biased articles. *American Family Physician.* September 1, 2011; 84(5): 489–490.

89 NAMS. NAMS Corporate Liaison Council. The Menopause Society. Accessed 12_ December, 2023. https://www.menopause.org/commercial-supporters/nams-corporate-liaison-council.

90 NAMS. About NAMS. Accessed December 12, 2023. https://www.menopause.org/About-NAMS.

91 Tatsioni A, Siontis GC, Ioannidis JP. Partisan perspectives in the medical literature: A study of high frequency editorialists favoring hormone replacement therapy. *Journal of General Internal Medicine.* September ; 25(9): 914–919. doi:10.1007/s11606-010-1360-7.

92 Bluming AZ, Hodis HN, Langer RD. 'Tis but a scratch: A critical review of the Women's Health Initiative evidence associating menopausal hormone therapy with the risk of breast cancer. *Menopause.* December 1, 2023; 30(12): 1241–1245. doi:10.1097/gme.0000000000002267.

93 Gannon L. *Women and aging; Transcending the myths.* Routledge; 1999.

94 Weissfeld JL, Liu W, Woods C, et al. Trends in oral and vaginally administered estrogen use among US women 50 years of age or older with commercial health insurance. *Menopause.* June 2018; 25(6): 611–614. doi:10.1097/gme.0000000000001054.

95 Hunter M, Lisha, N, Huang, A. Prescription of estrogen therapy and sedating medications in older women in a national ambulatory care sample. *Journal of the American Geriatric Society.* February 26, 2024. doi:10.1111/jgs.18844. Online ahead of print.

96 Grand View Research. Hormone replacement therapy market size, share & trend analysis by product (Estrogen & Progesterone Replacement Therapy), by route of administration, by disease type, by region, and segment forecasts, 2023–2030. Grand View Research. Accessed November 19, 2023. www.grandviewresearch.com/industry-analysis/hormone-replacement-therapy-market.

CONCLUSIONS

Mary Hunter

Conventional advertisements for many of the products mentioned in this book appear in printed literature, on television, and on the Internet. Women are typically portrayed as healthy, attractive, athletic, and able to make informed decisions, yet the advertisements contain an implicit warning: Conformation to the illustrated standard only results from using the product. This type of advertisement is easily recognized as a marketing message. Product claims might be fabricated, but it is clear that the generator of the message is the corporation that makes the product or the vendor that sells it.

In contrast, most marketing message origins are hidden, and many marketing messages are unconsciously perceived as established facts rather than marketing claims. As the movie title suggests, in our world of *everything everywhere all at once* we encounter marketing messages carefully crafted to shape our opinions. Most marketing messages (including those relating to political philosophies and science skepticism) are inserted into our uncritical minds so deftly that we fail to perceive the thought insertion, and we accept the messages as common sense. Marketing messages of this type, whether they promote a consumer product or lend credence to a point of view, exemplify third-party marketing.

Third-party Marketing, Including Ghostwriting

Third-party marketing messages appear to come from an impartial and objective source rather than from a corporation marketing a product. This marketing technique can involve utilizing a journalist, or imitating the role of one, to provide promotional messaging to media outlets as "news" coverage.[1] Marketer-generated print articles, audio segments, and video clips created to convey

DOI: 10.4324/9781003472711-8

marketing messages are ubiquitous. They are appreciated by cash-strapped and understaffed newspapers and radio and television stations struggling to produce enough content to justify their existence. Designed to be perceived as a newsworthy report of completed and valid research, marketer-supplied "news" is produced with high production values that lend the segment characteristics of a reliable news report. There is an entire industry devoted to creating and disseminating third-party marketing content.[2] Most of it is provided free to media outlets.

A typical example of a medical "news" report involves an interview with a spokesperson who reports a new "scientific" finding and speculates that the finding has implications for human health. The "news" finding may also have implications for increasing sales of a product used to prevent or treat a related condition. Although the report may appear to contain medically significant findings, it is subterfuge. Science reports of this type may or may not mention ongoing research or plans for future research to test specific hypotheses. Truly newsworthy research reports contain the words "as reported in [name of a peer-reviewed medical journal]."

Although third-party marketing might be used to promote a particular product or a class of products, it is also used to promote ideas, concepts, and beliefs consistent with corporate objectives. The belief that smoking cessation does not benefit long-term smokers is one example. This false third-party marketing message has given millions of smokers an excuse not to quit.

Third-party marketing messages are amplified by media coverage of activities within promotional networks such as those consisting of patient groups, consumer advocates, or professional societies. Public relations firms often direct these activities, lobbyists use them to influence legislation, and think tanks produce papers referencing them.

Ghostwriting is a form of third-party marketing that involves claiming a manuscript was authored by a prominent figure (e.g., a researcher in a medical specialty), rather than by the employees of a marketing firm contracted by a corporation. These manuscripts might be either academic research papers or opinion columns. The work of Adriane Fugh-Berman and her colleagues at PharmedOut, a project of the Georgetown University Medical Center in the US, demonstrated practical strategies for identifying ghostwritten materials, including examining and comparing the text of similar articles.[3] An objective of PharmedOut is to advance evidence-based prescribing by educating healthcare professionals about pharmaceutical marketing practices.[4]

Another project to educate healthcare professionals about marketing practices is the Drug Industry Documents Archive (DIDA) at the University of California San Francisco (UCSF).[5] This archive, accessible on a public website, contains an extensive collection of marketing documents, including documents related to ghostwriting. The documents include internal memos about communications between corporate employees, marketing firms, and medical professionals recruited as "authors." Many documents in the archives are discovery documents from lawsuits against corporations mentioned in this book.

A box of documents leaked by the cigarette manufacturer Brown & Williamson in 1994 was the start of a tobacco industry document collection that grew into the DIDA, now housed in the UCSF library.[6] The Brown & Williamson documents were used by researchers at UCSF to provide definitive proof that the tobacco industry hid their knowledge that nicotine was addictive and cigarettes caused cancer. UCSF research on the tobacco industry continues at the Center for Tobacco Control Research and Education (CTCRE), along with research on other corporate influences on health. Documents related to the pharmaceutical, sugar, chemical, and fossil fuel industries are also housed in the archives. The CTCRE holds an annual (virtual) workshop to train researchers to use the archives.[7]

The section of the archive featuring the promotion of opioids includes documents focused on the targeting of children and veterans.[8] Researchers have reported that sales slogans for opioids match those found in tobacco industry promotional materials. The collection has been used by academics, journalists, and filmmakers to increase public awareness of opioid marketing. It includes documents demonstrating how the marketing of opioids caused hundreds of thousands of patients in the US to turn to street drugs when their prescriptions were discontinued, or doses were reduced in response to the over-prescription of opioids. During 2023 and 2024, thousands of opioid documents were added to the archive monthly, and an estimated ten million more documents were yet to be added. Overall, the volume of materials in the DIDA is a testament to the enormity of impacts on public health resulting from third-party marketing.

Social Situations and Marketing

Most of the chapters in this book demonstrate that marketers expect consumers to buy specific products to help them meet social expectations. This helps explain the vast array of hair products at stores like Target. Marketing campaigns are tailored to address expectations related to age, gender, racial, and ethnic stereotypes. To make people want some iteration of whatever a corporation is selling, marketers take advantage of the social situations of their customers.

In her book *Situational Analysis*, Adele Clarke described a process for conducting qualitative analyses that researchers worldwide have found useful.[9] This process helps answer the basic question "What is going on?" In terms of marketing, the "situation" includes everything about a potential customer, whatever shapes her as a person. Let me restate that. The situation includes everything about what shapes a woman as a potential victim of a harmful product. A woman's life experiences, family and community, home and workplace, local and national politics, healthcare policies, and the histories of all these things are part of the situation.

Marketers consider multiple factors when designing a sales campaign, and a social scientist examining a marketing campaign might want to consider what the marketer has considered. In addition to examining the consumer and the marketer, the scientist would investigate the corporation. The situation of the corporation includes everything about its history and legal structure, the products it sells, and the way those products are marketed. Whether situational analysis is performed systematically, as described in Dr. Clarke's book, or the concept is used as a general reminder to look at *everything* one can think of that could possibly be important, considering the situation is critical.[9] Check out *Situational Analysis* if you are not already familiar with the theory and method. Making messy maps, a simple process explained in the book, is invaluable to a social scientist, especially at the beginning of a project.

Summaries of Marketing Strategies and Their Situations

In the first chapter, "The Stink of Clean," Beth Conway, describes household and personal care product messaging that plays on cultural, racial, and sexist notions about what it means to be clean. She cites social scientists who have argued that racial prejudice and misogyny shape the way household cleaning and personal care products are marketed to women, particularly in racist societies such as the United States (US).[10] The essay explains how marketing campaigns for these products tap into racial and gender stereotypes to leverage women's insecurities, and it shows how markets are segmented by the targeting of specific groups of women based on their ages and other demographic characteristics.

Fragrance allows marketers to connect with consumers silently and wordlessly, and while some consumers make conscious decisions to buy a product for its scent, others may be unaware of unconscious psychological and social cues that influence a purchasing decision. In either case, the consumer is not warned about or protected from the harms of toxic chemicals in household cleaning and personal care products, particularly those with fragrance ingredients.

Conway explores the exploitation of a perceived need to mask vaginal odor by marketers. She relates this phenomenon to misogynistic social cues and women's lack of knowledge about their bodies. Because vaginal douches, vulvar sprays, and the like are made with ingredients banned in many countries, they are not recommended by medical professionals, yet the use of these products is common in the US where they are marketed without regulation.

Conway critiques a near-total absence of regulation in the US of toxic chemicals in household cleaning and personal care products, and she compares this to the high degree of regulation of toxins in similar products across Europe and other high-income countries. The essay also addresses the improper classification of vaginal products as cosmetics, and the inadequate regulation of toxins in cosmetics.

The second chapter, "Tobacco Industry Corporate Malfeasance and Women's Rights Violations: Are Human Rights Mechanisms the Antidote?" by Kelsey Romeo-Stuppy, addresses a multinational corporate marketing campaign that comprises perhaps the most widespread and damaging threat to public health in history. The essay outlines how transnational tobacco corporations sell cigarettes in countries lacking legal protections for women consumers and workers. While sales of cigarettes have declined in the US because of public health efforts, the banning of cigarette advertising, and the imposition of tobacco taxes, a vast potential market of women smokers exists in the Global South. The same strategies used to market cigarettes to US women are being redeployed in countries where women do not yet smoke.

Transnational feminism addresses the gendered dimensions of injustices resulting from international commerce. In her introduction to *Gender and Global Justice*, Alison Jaggar noted that "the integration of the global economy has increased the sexualization of women."[11] She was specifically discussing women turning by economic necessity to sex work; however, her observation that globalization disrupts communities and impoverishes women is closely related to the consequences of marketing cigarettes. Globalization increases women's vulnerability to cigarette marketing messages that equate smoking with independence.

The marketing of cigarettes to women is a key example of how to sell a lethal and addictive product by associating its use with empowerment and social desirability. Marketing messages inviting US women to try cigarettes in the 1960s aligned with the emergence of second wave feminism. This was an era when televisions were brought into homes, cigarettes were advertised between programs, cigarette companies sponsored much of the programming, and cigarette product placement in programs proved to be an effective marketing strategy. Seeing prominent people smoking cigarettes proved to be as powerful a trigger for smokers, including smokers trying to quit, as advertisements. Advertising cigarettes on television, radio, and in magazines has been banned in the US since the early 1970s. Before the ban (which was signed by President Nixon in 1970 but was not enforceable until 1972), advertisements for thin, filtered cigarettes helped women smokers feel worldly, chic, sexy, and independent. Cigarette packaging designed to appeal to women reinforced the message that women are entitled to smoke with style.

Advertisements linking cigarette smoking to freedom, modernity, and empowerment, like those employed decades earlier in North America and Europe, are aired in the Global South on television screens, in movies, in magazines, on billboards, and on the Internet. The ads are meant to motivate uninitiated women to try cigarettes, and they are designed to remind current smokers that they would like another cigarette, right now. These ads violate women's human rights.

Romeo-Stuppy argues that failing to ban tobacco advertising is a human rights abuse and that women, and all beings with lungs, have the right to breathe air uncontaminated by cigarette smoke in the workplace and everywhere else. She argues convincingly that multinational collaboration, such as the World Health Organization (WHO) Framework Convention on Tobacco Control (FCTC), is needed to augment national tobacco-control policies to counter multinational tobacco corporations' intent to spread tobacco products throughout the world. While most countries are already party to the treaty, the US is not among them. Multinational tobacco companies, most of them based in the US, have $US billions at stake.

The third chapter, "Mother's Little Helpers and Opioids: Women, Addiction, and the Legacy of Arthur Sackler," like the chapter on tobacco, is about the marketing of incredibly addicting drugs. This essay illustrates that a simplistic and unsophisticated marketing strategy can be highly effective if a simple false claim (that a drug is not as addictive as people thought) is believed. "So this new [benzodiazepine or opioid] won't be a problem? That's great news!" The success of such a simple strategy says a lot about the gullibility of medical professionals regarding pharmaceutical product claims.

Although parts of the opioid epidemic story have been told in televised dramas and covered in news media, important aspects have been overlooked or underemphasized, and the drug epidemic continues to worsen. The promotion of benzodiazepines and opioids was included in this book, not because these drug classes are marketed primarily to women but because women become dependent on them more quickly than men, and women's lives are disproportionately affected when they experience addiction. In addition, Purdue's efforts to minimalize the addiction propensity of OxyContin and promote it for post-surgical pain, including pain following cesarean surgeries and other obstetric complications, led to high rates of opioid dependence in childbearing women. Some women long past their childbearing years have never recovered. Other women are still being exposed to opioids this way.

The marketing strategies used by Arthur Sackler to sell Librium and Valium were tactics imitated by his brothers to sell OxyContin. Dr. Sackler was among the earliest marketing professionals to engineer an early form of third-party marketing. He was among the first to manufacture a fake schema of doctors' endorsements for a pharmaceutical product, as in "Nine out of ten [people who should know] recommend [this product]." He published a free medical journal containing bogus research reports claiming that Librium and Valium, both highly addictive benzodiazepines, would not produce drug dependence. Arthur Sackler engineered a reward system for his own marketing efforts, tying his earnings to sales growth and profits, a system that anticipated similar programs created by his brothers to reward top Purdue detail representatives and prolific prescribers of OxyContin. Chain drugstores were rewarded for not questioning prescriber practices.[8]

Detail representatives are a direct marketing link between pharmaceutical companies and prescribers. When detail representatives saw evidence of rapid addiction contradicting the sales literature provided by Purdue, some of them became whistle-blowers. Much of the impetus for legal action in the US to end Purdue's fraudulent marketing of OxyContin resulted from the efforts of detail representatives who refused to comply with the company's instructions to lie about addiction propensity. Just as Big Tobacco has shifted cigarette marketing to untapped reservoirs of potential smokers in the Global South, Purdue has shifted much of its OxyContin marketing out of the US and is spreading the opioid epidemic to other parts of the globe.

The fourth chapter, "Under the Influence: Pharmaceutical Relationships and Their Impact on Endometriosis Care," outlines marketing tactics used by pharmaceutical companies to ensure that medical society treatment guidelines, such as those of the European Society of Human Reproduction and Embryology, mention their patented and costly products as first-line, definitive treatment. Heather Guidone's chapter on endometriosis drug marketing explores how corporations use industry partnerships to control treatment guidelines.

Gonadotropin-releasing hormone (GnRH) analogs can be useful for treating pain associated with endometriosis; however, they are not curative, and they are associated with high rates of significant side effects, including depression and osteoporosis. GnRH analogs are profitable for pharmaceutical corporations. Other drugs with efficacy in treating endometriosis pain, such as progestins and non-steroidal anti-inflammatory drugs, are underemphasized in treatment guidelines despite the fact that they are less expensive and have fewer side effects. When GnRH analogs are promoted as state-of-the art definitive treatment, despite evidence that expert surgery may be more appropriate in many cases, avoidance or delay of surgery potentially squanders a patient's fertility and prolongs symptoms.

Guidone's chapter illustrates common techniques used by drug companies to create a hegemonic discourse and set of conditions favoring their products. Creating such a discourse is accomplished by creating a web of partnerships among a variety of influential entities. The word "web" is used here rather than the word "network," because creating a web connotes connivance and collusion. This essay illustrates in detail how a web of partnerships works to influence endometriosis treatment and promote GnRH analogs.

Guidone describes the numerous parties involved in this web, including patient advocacy groups, participants in roundtables, professional society guideline advisory boards, joint-professional working groups, and politicians able to vote on relevant legislation and make budget decisions. The pharmaceutical corporations mentioned in this chapter and many others have been reported to hire lobbyists and ghostwriting firms, pay so-called "kickbacks" to individual physicians, and endow fellowships and sponsor research projects in exchange for reports with findings favoring their drugs. These parties work in concert to support a discourse useful in promoting GnRH analogs as superior to other treatments, including surgery. By cultivating webs of partnerships, marketers ensure that costly drugs remain profitable. Tactics used to control the content of professional society guidelines outlined by Guidone provide a blueprint for studying this phenomenon in other industries.

The fifth chapter, a content analysis and theoretical essay by Anna Kubovski entitled "Menstruation Repression Discourse in Advertisements: An Ecofeminist Investigation," contributes a marketing perspective to menstrual cycle studies literature. This body of literature connects numerous disciplines, including nursing and medicine, health policy, global health, psychology, sociology, social justice, education, law, and feminist studies, including ecofeminism.[12] Although her chapter centers primarily on the psychological impact of advertisements for products used to contain menstrual blood, Kubovski also writes about potential adverse health and environmental consequences associated with disposable pads and tampons. It is useful to consider these issues in a global context.

In the Global South, persistent discrimination against menstruators in patriarchal societies leaves many girls, women, and gender-diverse people without access to disposable pads and tampons.[13] Menstrual discrimination contributes to inadequate educational opportunities and underemployment, resulting in poverty and contributing to the incidence of child marriage. Just as greater access to these products is pursued in the Global South, public health activists in more affluent countries work to ensure that cost does not limit access to pads and tampons and contribute to absence from school or work.

The use of disposable pads and tampons is increasing across the globe, and while this has mostly positive consequences for individuals, it has a decidedly negative impact on the environment. The language and conceptual framing of containment of menstrual blood employed by disposable menstrual product marketers have created a near-universal assumption that these products are necessary for the health and well-being of women, and advertisements continually reinforce this assumption.

One might question whether this assumption is mutable, and there are additional questions to answer. Do women require disposable menstrual products to thrive in society? What are the potential consequences of efforts to expand markets for disposable products throughout the Global South? Does increasing access to disposable products (in any country or society) hamper efforts to increase the utilization of reusable menstrual products? Are women everywhere, and is the planet best served by efforts to increase access to reusable menstrual cups and absorbent underwear? What are the potential barriers to efforts to promote reusable products (e.g., cultural, social, economic, or health-related)? What can be done to mitigate the environmental impact of both disposable and reusable products?

All the marketing techniques discussed in previous essays are illustrated in the sixth chapter, "Hot and Bothered by the Menopause Industry." Leveraging personal and social insecurities, menopausal hormone therapy (HT) marketing typically incorporates imagery suggesting that hormone pills, patches, and creams help women preserve or improve their personal appeal and social positions. It gives users the sense that they can control the ravages of time, and that they will look and perform better than women who don't use HT.[14,15] Long-term users believe that HT has helped keep them healthy, and that it will continue to keep them healthy. They resist quitting when the risks of diseases associated with long-term HT outweigh potential benefits.

A key HT marketing strategy is providing misinformation about risk and creating doubt about risk information.[15] Marketers ensure that sources of risk information are discounted as unreliable (e.g., the Women's Health Initiative in the US and the Million Women Study in the UK), and confusion resulting from the obfuscation of risk information interferes with health-related decision-making. Moreover, product benefits are purported to "cancel out" potential risks.

A tendency to seek out or interpret information in a way that reinforces one's existing beliefs is known as "confirmation bias." Confirmation bias intensifies marketing messages about product benefits, and it enables women to disregard risk evidence published by competent and ethical scientists. The Internet is the perfect place to look for claims of HT benefits that can be used to cancel out any lingering risk concerns. The marketing claim that HT keeps skin looking young has been particularly effective.

Marketers place promotional messaging in professional medical journal articles and medical "news" stories in various media, and they find famous women with great skin to provide endorsements for estrogen in magazine articles, books, and on television. HT marketing continues to suggest that estrogen improves the skin, and ghostwritten articles, particularly those citing Mark Brincat, MD, still appear (as citations) in medical journals. Forty-one documents in the UCSF Drug Industry Document archive connect Mark Brincat with this ghostwriting effort funded primarily by Wyeth-Ayerst Pharmaceuticals.[16] (Type "Brincat" into the search box to find the 41 articles; 202 documents are presented when the words "estrogen and skin" are typed into the search box.)

In the menopause industry, as in the endometriosis drug industry, marketers create webs of influence among industry partners to manipulate treatment guidelines to favor their products. Product dependence is reinforced, and sales are sustained, when products are available from a variety of sources, despite limited regulatory interference with distribution channels. The availability of HT in the form of compounded hormones assures continued access should long-term users be denied ongoing prescriptions from conscientious providers.

The promotion of HT perfectly illustrates "medicalization," a social phenomenon and strategy used by pharmaceutical corporations to promote products for conditions that can reasonably be considered normal aspects of human existence.

After decades of deceptive and spectacularly effective marketing, much of society views menopause as an illness, medicalizing the aging of women is taken for granted, and the menopause industry continues to grow harming increasing numbers of older women.

Final Thoughts

Ignoring good science, marketers deny product risks and make claims for false benefits. To sell household cleaning and personal care products, cigarettes, and drugs, corporate marketers leverage a need for social acceptance and a universal desire to maintain control of one's body and life circumstances. Strategies to sell anti-anxiety agents and painkillers take advantage of psychological and physical pain while offering the hope of regaining a lost sense of well-being.

All but one of the marketing campaigns we examined take advantage of a woman's desire to feel well and stay healthy. Although tobacco was once marketed using claims of health benefits, cigarette smoking is no longer promoted as health enhancement. This suggests that when public health advocates challenge corporate marketing practices, change is possible.

Notes

1 Farsetta D. Public Relations and Advertising. In: Wiist W, Ed. *The bottom line or public health*. Oxford University Press; 2010: 118–120.

2 Adgate B. Advertising In Reliable News Sources Provides Stronger Brand Effectiveness. *Forbes*. 11_3_21 ed: Forbes; 2021.

3 Fugh-Berman A. The Haunting of Medical Journals: How Gostwriting Sold "HRT". *PLoS Medicine*. September 2010; 7(9): e1000335. doi:10.1371/journal.pmed. 1000335.

4 PharmedOut. Georgetown University Medical Center. https://sites.google.com/ georgetown.edu/pharmedout.

5 Drug Industry Documents. University of California San Francisco Library. www. industrydocuments.ucsf.edu/drug.

6 Chur E. Faculty Spotlight: Stanton Glantz, PhD. UCSF. Accessed January 17, 2024. https://ucsfhealthcardiology.ucsf.edu/facstaff/spotlight/glantz.

7 Education CfTCRa. Annual Tobacco and Other Industries Documents Workshop. UCSF. Accessed January 17, 2024. https://tobacco.ucsf.edu/annual-tobacco-and-other-industries-documents-workshop.

8 Buller R. Corporate Strategy, National Tragedy. *UCSF Magazine*. Winter 2024.

9 Clarke A. *Situational analysis: Grounded theory after the postmodern turn*. Sage; 2005: xli.

10 Berthold D. Tidy Whiteness: A Genealogy of Race, Purity, and Hygiene. *Ethics and the Environment*. 2010; 15(1): 1–26.

11 Jaggar AM. *Gender and global justice*. Polity; 2014: x.

12 Warren K, Erkal N. *Ecofeminism : Women, culture, nature*. Indiana University Press; 1997: xvi.

13 Paudel R. *Dignified menstruation: The dignity of menstruators throughout their life Cycle*. Kathmandu Publication; 2020.

14 Hunter MM, Huang AJ, Wallhagen MI. "I'm Going to Stay Young": Belief in Anti-aging Efficacy of Menopausal Hormone Therapy Drives Prolonged Use Despite Medical Risks. *PloS one*. 2020; 15(5): e0233703. doi:10.1371/journal.pone.0233703.

15 Hunter MM. Hormone Therapy Decision Making in Older Women. Doctoral. University of California San Francisco. Accessed ISBN 978043876035. https://escholarship.org/uc/item/70v4k4b2.

16 Brincat search. Drug Industry Documents. UCSF Library. Accessed January 14, 2024. www.industrydocuments.ucsf.edu/drug/results/#q=Brincat&h=%7B%22hide Duplicates%22%3Afalse%2C%22hideFolders%22%3Atrue%7D&subsite=drug&c ache=true&count=41.

INDEX

Printed in the United States
by Baker & Taylor Publisher Services

Printed in the United States
by Baker & Taylor Publisher Services